MEN AND WOMEN OF VILCABAMBA:
HEALTHY, ROBUST, ACTIVE,
AND 100+ YEARS OLD.

Micaela Quezada, 104, a virgin and proud of it.
But the villagers say she might still get married
some day.

Manuel Ramon, 110, doesn't know the meaning
of the word "retirement." He works in the field
every day of the week except Sunday.

Miguel Carpio, 127, lives in a bare little house
and behaves with the courtesy and grace of a
philosopher-king.

Gabriel Erazo, a lusty 132 years old, keeps alive
the dream of a great love in years to come—and
propositioned the author unabashedly.

Los Viejos

Secrets of Long Life
from the Sacred Valley

by
Grace Halsell

BANTAM BOOKS · TORONTO · NEW YORK · LONDON

*This low-priced Bantam Book
has been completely reset in a type face
designed for easy reading, and was printed
from new plates. It contains the complete
text of the original hard-cover edition.*
NOT ONE WORD HAS BEEN OMITTED.

RL 8, IL 8+

LOS VIEJOS
*A Bantam Book | published by arrangement with
Rodale Press, Inc.*

PRINTING HISTORY
*Rodale Press edition published July 1976
2nd printing .... December 1976
Bantam edition | July 1978*

ISBN 0-553-10729-1

Published simultaneously in the United States and Canada

---

*Bantam Books are published by Bantam Books, Inc. Its trade-
mark, consisting of the words "Bantam Books" and the por-
trayal of a bantam, is registered in the United States Patent
Office and in other countries. Marca Registrada. Bantam
Books, Inc., 666 Fifth Avenue, New York, New York 10019.*

PRINTED IN THE UNITED STATES OF AMERICA

Contents

Preface

One of our oldest dreams is to live in a perfect garden, a Shangri-la where you never show your wrinkles or grow decrepit—even if you live to 132.

For the past three years I have been researching the mystery, and the marvel, of adding years to our lives.

As part of this research, I lived for a year in a country in South America, a country—Ecuador—little known to North Americans. I stayed for the most part in the village of Vilcabamba, that lies hidden behind a majestic range of mountains, some of the tallest and most inspiring in all of the world. And from this village, I went out into areas of utter isolation to live in simple huts with the men and women who are the longest living people of the western hemisphere.

I lived in the huts of Gabriel Erazo, Manuel Carpio, Gabriel Sanchez, Manuel Ramon, and Micaela Quezada, who claim they are 132, 127, 113, 110 and 104, respectively.

Ecuadorian doctors believe that those ages are correct, and they can show you baptismal records that definitely "prove" certain ages.

At half their ages, I could not keep up with them. I can testify: they are *very old*, and more important, they are active—alive and *loving* people.

In 1974, while I was living in the village of Vilcabamba, a team of American medical experts came to learn the "secrets" of the Old People's longevity. Ironically, the U.S. doctors all fell ill in Vilcabamba. They found living conditions deplorable. One doctor was stricken with the malady known as "sleeping sickness" and the others became ill because they could not tolerate the food or the water. Over the years the Old People had become immune to certain bacteria.

In Vilcabamba, I came to know men and women who are without things, who are stripped down to their basic selves. I was forced to examine them as human beings, uniquely individual and autonomous.

In Washington, D.C., I often do not see the personality, the man—but rather his $250 suit, or his impressive title.

While working for President Johnson in the White House, I had come to know men with impressive titles and big salaries who had no awareness of themselves, no sense of their own personalities.

Also, I have watched one executive friend run— without looking—toward material goals. He once admitted, "If I stop, I fear that I will encounter *me*. And I don't want to do that, I'm afraid."

And this was true with some of the doctors who came to the Sacred Valley.

I asked each of the American doctors: Where did we come from? Why are we here? Where are we going? These "Ultimate Questions," as they are called, were formulated by the Hebrews and the Greeks two or three millennia ago. And the search for answers to these questions has provided the world with its great religions. None of the doctors could answer, or at least none would verbalize *any* answer. One doctor, Harold Elrick of California, said, "Listen, I've been too busy becoming a doctor. I have not had *time* to think about such questions."

But each of the Old People had taken the time to face the ultimate questions, and each had an answer ready—as if he or she had been waiting for the past 50 years for me to pop that particular question.

They did not know a lot about science or our modern "facts," but they knew that the greatest wisdom is to know yourself.

Their statements on the "meaning" of life were

the equivalent of what Socrates or Unamuno might have said.

And they had a great philosopher's modesty. When Señor Ramon told me he had lived 110 years, he added, "To live—is to learn to die," and he said it with full knowledge of the limitations of any man.

For me, coming to know them was a spiritual experience. They have blessed my life—and I am eager to share some of these "blessings" with you.

Grace Halsell
Washington, D.C. 1976

Los Viejos

1

Vilcabamba

In 1974 I went to the small, isolated village of Vilcabamba in the rugged Andean mountain terrain of southern Ecuador to live with the oldest people in the western hemisphere.

My purpose was a simple one: I wanted to find out whether there was an answer to the fears of old age nurtured by men and women in our urban, industrial world—fears of becoming helpless and useless, of a total dependence on others, of decrepitude and despair. I had read extensively of flourishing centenarians in Russia, Hunza and Ecuador, and I started with Ecuador, fully expecting at a later time to visit the Abkhasians in Russia and the Hunzas in Pakistan. But in Ecuador I discovered some answers, some clues, some intimations which prompted me to write solely about the long-living people in our own hemisphere.

They became my heroes. Their simplicity, the beauty of their lives became patterns for me to emulate. I could not have met any young person, no matter how valiant, how knowledgeable, who inspired me as the people of Vilcabamba.

As we add years to our lives, we realize anew that the unexamined life is not worth leading. I wanted to study what growing old means in my own personal life. Aging is a singular distinction in a time when distinctions are being desperately obliterated. Further, I yearned to pay tribute to my father, who lived to the age of 96, and my mother, the most remarkable man and woman I have known, who showed me the best examples of courage and happiness, the qualities that I most admire. Today my mother, 83, is a lively, energetic, beautiful person. She radiates a hope and zest for today and tomorrow. In her, I see that growing old means a growing appreciation for love—given and received.

At sixty, seventy and eighty, my father, who was born in Texas in 1860, was strong, with muscles few men in their twenties or thirties have. He credited his strength to long years of outdoor life, many days on horseback, often for as much as 20 hours, enduring in the saddle and on foot the rigors of bitter winters and torrid summers.

He was always a happy, energetic man. One who would make you glad you knew him.

My father's love for my mother and her love for him have always been an unquestioned feature of my dreams and my reality. It was never a synthetic "love" or a pretense for the children. Each had earned the other's love, and it was as real as their heartbeat, as genuine as breath.

Because, perhaps, of my love for my aged father, I easily identified with the long-living people of Vilcabamba. There were other reasons, as well. In the 1960s, I had lived for three years in neighboring Peru, and also I have lived in Mexico, and have always felt that my heart's home lies somewhere south of the border.

So, when I decided to go live among the centenarians, I located Vilcabamba on a map of Ecuador, and started out—travelling alone.

Beginning with the year I turned 18, I have always travelled the world alone. And I have been warned, you may get *taken in* and indeed I have, but always by kind-hearted people.

In a career that has embraced daily journalism, the writing of numerous magazine articles and books, I have always gone to other lands with one idea: to meet people and come to know them. I learn to sing their songs, dance their jigs, eat their food. I try to stay in their homes, to be one among the people in whose land I am living.

Before going to Vilcabamba I knew, however, that within a few months' time a team of American doctors would come to the village to make scientific studies of the long-living people. Meanwhile, I wanted to go on my own, asking them to take me in—to let me be a part of their circle of loved ones.

In this manner, I came to know men and women who were not only very old—*viejos*, as they are called in their native Spanish language—but also individuals with strong personalities, a well-founded sense of their own identities, and a charming innocence about their own uniqueness.

Visitors to Vilcabamba claim there is "something special" about the valley, and yet the *viejos* are in many respects like millions of dirt-poor country folk: hardworking, uncomplicated and relatively serene.

Through stern physical labor they have earned for themselves a self-respect and sense of fulfillment missing in many urban lives. They are as one with the soil, as native to the earth as a seed of corn. Nature's cycle governs their lives, from the green promise of spring to the mature ripeness of autumn. Age has mellowed and enriched them. Modern victims of the myriad distractions and demands of our industrial society might conclude that the *viejos* are bored with the profound simplicity of their lives. But it is not true. They are renewed by the changing seasons, the process of growth in which they participate as energetic allies.

They live hard, sparse lives, and in earthly goods, they are well below the poverty line. But they have accumulated huge reserves of goodwill. They seem to have been bred for a special brand of gentility, a freedom from the corrosive effects of hatred, an immunity to violence.

I came to know them as only one can who goes in

need. I needed them to "take me in," to provide a place for me to sleep, to provide food for me to eat, to provide answers for my own search of how to live through one's last years with dignity, spirit and fortitude. I lived in their primitive huts, with their dirt floors, and I slept on their beds of rough-hewn wooden boards. I ate their boiled corn called *mote*, and I listened endlessly to their stories of romance and love and the manner in which they give a meaning to their lives.

They know nothing of politics. The economics of their existence is measured in what they earn to feed and clothe themselves. Their large dramas center on affairs of the human heart.

Manuel Ramon at a reported 110 had a face radiating an almost animal-like force. When I felt his strong biceps and praised his ability to climb mountains I could not ascend and go to work from sunup to sunset in a field of maize, he bowed his head shyly, and confessed in his modest way: "It is no great thing I do."

Señora Mariana Tolédo had never been to a beauty salon, never used lipstick, powder or rouge. But time had not robbed her of an inner radiance and her smile suggested that her husband found her an attractive mate. She was thin, with acute faculties, good vision, good hearing, a clear mind and an excellent memory. She was independent, even tempered, possessed of a lively humor and found it easy to laugh. She had never owned a clock ("I don't need it," she said), had never seen TV or listened to a radio.

Mariana Herrera and I talked about airplanes (she had heard of them but never saw one) and flights to the moon (she refused to believe that a man could walk on the moon). Then, with an unabashed simplicity, she talked about the happiness that comes to a woman when she lies in the arms of a man she loves. In her ninety-two years, she said, with an earthy directness that was too natural to doubt, nothing had equalled that quiet sense of joy and well-being.

Micaela Quezada, 104, slender and erect in a floor-length black dress with a shawl draped around her head, punctuated her words with theatrical gestures: "I had two sisters who married men who beat them, gave them black eyes, *ojos negros*," she claimed. Not wanting to subject herself to such indignities, she had all of her long years remained a virgin. She told this quite proudly, as another woman might boast of owning a Pucci original or a mink.

Gabriel Sanchez said matter-of-factly, "I am 113." He continues to climb the steep el Chaupi mountain and work all day with his crude hoe or *lampa*, cultivating a small plot of ground. He called me "*doctorita*," little doctor, and sometimes "*Nenita*," little one, and made me feel my life had just begun.

None of the *viejos* wore glasses or had hearing aids. Few of them needed a cane or crutch to help him or her walk. And none of them, as far as I was able to determine, ever suffered fractured bones. Dr. Richard Mazess, a University of Wisconsin anthropologist specializing in the study of calcium contents in bones, made a cursory study of the *viejos* in 1974. "I saw no evidence of fractures," he said. "They have good muscle structure. Also, I saw no apparent spinal curvature as you find in the older population of the United States. They are in good general health—and they are *active*, that's for sure. They are able to do for themselves, maintain themselves."

Dr. Mazess added, "If I could draw one conclusion it would be that parts of our body—our arms, our legs —must be kept in good working order if we want to avoid fracture. Here again, the old adage works: *use it or lose it.*"

The *viejos* had fit bodies, but their main concern had been the human heart. Their society seemed to be oriented toward the mystical, the religious, the romantic. Ours seemed to be oriented toward the scientific, the practical, and an empirical faith in "the survival of the fittest." But this begs the question because it does not tell us what fitness is for. It does not remind us that what is new is not necessarily what is good. Nor does it suggest to us what human destiny ought to be.

The *viejos* all kept romantic illusions, *amor* gave spirit to their lives. Gabriel Erazo composed poetry, and when we would take a walk at sunset he would quote his verses to me, leaving me feeling soft and vulnerable. "I am 132," he told me, and at the same moment he said he still had desires, *ganas,* to make love to a woman, that he felt this desire as strongly as he did when he was twenty. Medical science may have doubts about Gabriel's claim, but Gabriel certainly didn't.

Visitors to this secluded habitat, which is known as Sacred Valley, have yearned to discover if the people of Vilcabamba have a simple secret for longevity. It was only reasonable to assume that they must be doing something right in contrast to our own mode of living. In our urban, fast-paced, fast-food, noisy, cluttered environment, almost every day one hears of a friend or a friend of a friend who has dropped dead from a heart attack. The disease appears to be reaching younger people, to men in their 40s and even in their 30s. And like everything else in this and other advanced societies, the women are catching up with the men.

Kenneth H. Cooper, M.D., who designed a heart-strengthening exercise program for the United States Air Force and authored the best-selling book *Aerobics* detailing his regimen, reports that "death from heart disease in young American women is the highest of any country in the world."

The longevity of American men ranks 17th and that of American women ranks tenth among the major nations of the world. Calling heart disease "a national disaster," Dr. Cooper said the malady has become the Nation's Number One health problem. Every year nearly a million Americans die from heart and blood vessel disease—a mortality rate higher than that of any other country. Many of these victims are half the age of the *viejos.* Why is this? What might be different or special about the village? The minerals in the soil? The diet? The *viejos'* attachment to the land, which they work with their hands until beckoned by death?

Could it be the genetic factor? The Vilcabamba enclave of centenarians pose a fascinating puzzle for science: How is it that a tiny group of men and women have managed to survive far longer than most people in our society?

Doctors who have visited there have given us only intriguing hints that there must be "something special" about the valley. Most likely, it is not a single, distinctive, identifiable factor that contributes toward longevity and good health, but a complex combination of many factors.

A United States doctor, Eugene H. Payne, wrote a 1954 *Reader's Digest* article in which he stated he had found little or no evidence of cardiac or circulatory diseases in the area. Another visitor, Albert B. Kramer, writing in a 1959 issue of *Prevention*, reported he suffered a cardiac condition but after a short visit to the province, he said, "I felt better than I could ever remember." He rhapsodized over the lush forest growth at altitudes where one would normally expect barren slopes. "Can you imagine," he asked, "strawberries growing next to banana plants, coffee thriving in the shade of apple trees, barley and sugar cane growing side by side?" He was quite willing to accept that "something special" distinguished the province. "Perhaps that 'something' that is so good for the heart is the same 'something' that so strangely favors plant life," he wrote.

Dr. Miguel Salvador, a Quito cardiologist with an expansive personality, who has lived in the United States as well as Paris, first became interested in Vilcabamba after hearing reports that residents there never suffered heart attacks. An Ecuadorian government agency appointed the cardiologist to take specialists into Vilcabamba for a major research study of the area. In 1969, Dr. Salvador, with a team of Ecuadorian doctors, made a survey of 340 persons of all ages selected at random from Vilcabamba's total population. They found the general standard of fitness among the old "amazing," an unprofessional but plainly apt description. Almost all were free of serious illness. The valley, the doctors concluded, was indeed a natural island of immunity to the physical and perhaps psychological problems that shorten lives elsewhere.

"We had gone there to study heart conditions," Dr. Salvador explained. "And it was while we were making our heart studies that we learned for the first time, almost accidentally, you might say, that there were so many old people. One out of six persons in the village was over the age of 65, twice the average for the United States and Canada, for example, and five times the figure for the rest of Ecuador."

Dr. Salvador added, "We had to believe their ages, because of their accounts, reports and narrations, as well as the ages of their children and grandchildren. I was impressed, however, not because people were living to be more than 100, but because they were so active, with minds and bodies you'd expect in men and women who were 60 or 70." In the comparatively few cases of heart disease that did occur in the valley, Dr. Salvador said, the symptoms were not felt and treatment was "not required."

"When I went there in 1969 I found that there were victims of heart attacks, but that some victims showed no symptoms of having had an attack," Dr. Salvador explained. "Thus, if they did not feel that they were ill, they were, for all practical purposes, well and healthy. They carried on lives that were absolutely normal. It must be the same as the Hunzas in Pakistan where some have suffered heart attacks, but they feel as they would without the symptoms. One might feel very well, despite the lesion or injury."

A 1971 census identified nine centenarians in a total population of 819 people. Dr. Alexander Leaf, chief of medical services, Massachusetts General Hospital, Boston, observed that, "While extrapolation on the basis of this small village is not justifiable, the figures do represent a rate of 1,100 per 100,000 population, obviously an exceptional situation when compared with the U.S. rate of only three centenarians per 100,000 population."

While in Vilcabamba Dr. Leaf, the other American doctors and I spent long painstaking hours studying baptismal records kept by the local Catholic church.

The ledger, as large as your outstretched arms and as thick as a couple of Manhattan telephone directories, contained hundreds of names written in flourishing script by *padres*, many of whom had come from Spain to serve in the isolated village.

I was a little awed by the ancient church book, and also by the fact that the present priest had allowed us to take the ancient records, now beginning to fade and perish with age, out into the sunshine in order to photograph certain pages, containing names of the *viejos* we had come to know.

We found no baptismal records for Vilcabamba's alleged oldest citizens, Gabriel Erazo and Miguel Carpio. But one of Carpio's daughters had a baptismal record that documents her age at 86.

Several *viejos*, however, whose advanced ages were documented, told us they remembered when they were quite young that Carpio already was grown.

We did find information on a José Miguel Carpio, a younger brother of Miguel. And, we learned that this José Miguel Carpio was the fifth child born after Miguel Carpio.

The baptismal record shows that José was born in 1874.

We then figured that allowing two years between the birth of the five, Miguel Carpio would have been born about ten years after José Carpio, in other words about 1864. This would then make Miguel's age about 110 in the year of 1974, when we were making our investigation.

We found it most frustrating to hear Carpio tell us he was 127, and then, on our own, come up with a figure of *only* 110.

We finally concluded: the *viejos* may not know their exact ages, but in all cases they are very old and more important, they are remarkable, active people.

Dr. Leaf also visited two other pockets of longevity, the district known as Abkhazia in the Caucasus moun-

tains of Russia, and Hunza in the Karakoram range of
Pakistan, on the borders of Afganistan and China. The
men and women of Hunza have received a great deal
of worldwide attention because of their diet of vegetables, grains and fruits, especially apricots. Eaten
fresh in the summer, dried in the sun for the long winter, the apricot is a staple in Hunza, much as rice is in
other parts of the world.

The Russians have given much publicity to their
long-living people, but, unfortunately, little has been
subject to the scrutiny and verification of outsiders.
The Soviet press announced on September 2, 1973,
that the oldest known human being, Shirali Mislimov,
a resident of Barzavu, a village in Soviet Azerbaid-
zhan, had died at 168. No scientific reports explained
how he managed to live to such an extraordinary age.
Most experts in gerontology seriously doubt the Rus-
sian claim.

Province officials in Loja, with no real regard for the
welfare of the *viejos*, have been promoting the Sacred
Valley as a tourist resort, much in the same way one
might publicize recreational delights of a Disneyland
or Coney Island.

Up until 1974, however, they had not succeeded in
making many changes. And the doctors, hippies, jour-
nalists and heart sufferers who visited the valley made
little concrete difference, at least in outward appearance. There was still no plumbing, electricity, tele-
phones, newspapers, restaurants, hotels, TV, or radios.

There was one big improvement, however. The 30-
mile winding, mountainous dirt road from Loja was
being widened and turned into an all-weather asphalt
route. Dr. Salvador viewed the development darkly.
Once, as we bounced along in a jeep over the
road, he remarked, resignedly, "I wonder how long
will it take 'civilization' to get to Vilcabamba—and to
spoil it forever?"

Already, I could see the vast difference between the
lifestyle of the *viejos* and their descendants. The young
people do not want to get up at 5 A.M., to struggle up a
mountain, to work in the fields. They like to lounge

about in the village. And play nickelodeons and buy sweets that become so addictive. I sat in front of a general store in the village, and watched school children clutching pennies to buy ice cream and sugary colas and candy bars. Unwittingly they were lopping off years of their lives by indulging in the packaged sweets that our "modern" civilization has introduced to them.

The *viejos*, on the other hand, had reached longevity and maintained good health on a strict regime, their own do-it-yourself recipe.

Dr. Salvador and Dr. Leaf and other medical experts were aware of the rich irony involved in their investigation of the *viejos* who had lived to their remarkable old age without ever having had the benefit of a medical checkup or a drugstore prescription. Like ancient gnarled oak trees, they had made it on their own, aided by the sun, wind, rain and qualities of the human body and the heart, about which people, including doctors, apparently can only conjecture with any assurance.

The doctors knew that their investigations would be disruptive to the *viejos*' quiet life, and yet the studies were being done in the name of progress and with the hope they would be beneficial to countless others.

By the time the doctors arrived I felt like a native of Vilcabamba. I knew many of the families both in the village, and in the outlying mountains. I had adapted myself to their diet and to the custom of sleeping in their dirt-floor huts, on a hard board that merely extended from a wall, and, with blankets, served as a bed.

Moreover, I spoke Spanish, enabling me to serve as an interpreter for Dr. Leaf and other American doctors. Also, I have always wished that I could be a nurse, and I now had the opportunity to act as a doctor's assistant, or, as we now call it, a paramedical worker.

My objectives, however, were quite different from the doctors. I was not especially interested in blood pressure, heartbeat and urine analysis, but rather in attitude, motivations, lifestyle, philosophy, outlook and degree of happiness.

While we had our different goals, the doctors and I had one common goal. We were interested in knowing if factors common to exceptional longevity could be identified, and if by studying people who reach unusual old age without debility and senility we could shed light on how to prevent these conditions in our own population. We wondered if we could extract from the *viejos* neat and precise recipes for long, active and useful lives.

Americans have become increasingly concerned about how to remain useful and contented because of what one sociologist has called the "truly astonishing population revolution in America." In short, the lengthening of the life span in our population has made aging an issue of national concern.

In 1900 only four percent of the population was over 65, but today that figure has risen to ten percent, or 21 million people over 65. Diseases such as diphtheria or tuberculosis that once killed off many people before they passed middle age have slowly come under control; more and more people survive into their 60s and 70s.

By 2005, when the generation of the postwar baby boom reaches retirement age, some experts estimate, almost a quarter of the population will be 65 years and over. Old age has become a major medical preoccupation, and indeed, a preoccupation with many of us who do not worry about death so much as learning how to stay active and alert—for as long as we live.

The little we know about aging does not fully explain the variations—why some grow old in agony and bitterness, others with fortitude and beauty. We do not understand the factors that produce an energetic, alert and happy person at ninety and a debilitated, senile and unhappy one at sixty.

The experts in gerontology still wrestle with mysteries, riddles, enigmas of the human body, much as philosophers and psychologists still grope for answers to questions prompted by the human experience.

The historical record assures us that exceptional age does not automatically invite feebleness or decrepitude. It does not necessarily consign you to a limbo of uselessness. We admire the active, productive life of a Verdi, Voltaire, Hugo, Michelangelo, Picasso, Casals, Toscanini, Cervantes, Goethe, Tennyson, Wells, Shaw, Sophocles, Santayana, Colette and Grandma Moses, to name a few. The list affirms that some of our greatest musicians, writers, painters, poets reached their peaks well after our so-called retirement age.

In 1974 there were about 13,000 Americans over the age of 100, according to the Social Security Administration. Some were vigorous and alert, others withered and frail. In many ways, the traditional attitude of unhappy resignation toward old age has begun to change. Dr. Bernard Strehler of Los Angeles, president of the Association for the Advancement of Aging Research, said, "People generally accept that it is becoming possible to live much longer and healthier lives."

We are now accepting the notion that it is not "un-American" in this young nation of ours to grow old. We have always known about pediatrics, but only now are we learning about geriatrics, the study of the diseases of old age, and gerontology, the study of the aging process.

One might define aging as growing old. But then what is that? There is, for instance, no quantitative test that allows the physician to distinguish whether a patient is chronologically old or has aged more rapidly and is physiologically old.

"Unlike the annual rings in a tree," Dr. Leaf has explained, "nothing in the human body allows for accurate determination of age."

We have huge laboratories, great technology and the most modern of medical measuring devices, but we learn how to grow old not so much from theories as from examples of lives—lives as they are lived, in as common-as-the-bread-we-eat, ordinary, everyday, yet often heroic manner.

Some experts in aging look for a big "breakthrough," some spectacular discovery in science that will allow us to live—"forever." But most of us are not concerned with "forever" so much as we are interested in learning how to stay active and useful and happy, let's say up to 100. I went to learn from the *viejos*, because they had lived longer than any other known group in this western hemisphere. And most important, they are still working, and loving and lovable, and—what pleases me most of all—they spend a lot of their time *laughing*.

2

Genetics

Many old persons whose forebears lived to unusually ripe old ages often jestingly claim that the first rule for longevity is to make a careful selection of your parents.

In my own case, I feel lucky to have been born of good, healthy, long-living parents. But if I live to well past four score and ten, I will not know whether to credit the genes my parents bequeathed me or the diet they fed me, the work and exercise patterns they helped me establish, or the good, positive thoughts they encouraged me to entertain. I feel lucky not so much because of my genes (I know little about them) but because I grew up on the plains of Texas where I had space and fresh air, and a remarkably plain and wholesome diet. We had fresh fruit and vegetables from our garden and fresh milk and butter from our cow. The food we ate was almost always natural food. And my parents knew how to live a long and happy life. I would not want to disparage the role of my parents, in genetic or practical terms; they set good examples. But I cannot, in good conscience and in fealty to the facts, discount my own role, the kind of environment in which I grew up, and the lessons I learned from the natural elements that blessed me.

Accordingly, I came away from my stay in Vilcabamba convinced that the genetic factor, in itself, may or may not have added a few years to the lives of the *viejos*, just as it may or may not add years to your life or mine.

This largely remains a matter of conjecture, for, it seems to me, and to many others, that heredity and environment are complementary factors, difficult, if not impossible, to assign separate and precise values in the growth and development of any organism.

Perhaps the point can best be made if you were to imagine yourself a native of Vilcabamba, born of parents who lived into their 90s or beyond. However, you decide to leave the peaceful valley and move to a large, cluttered, polluted city, such as New York, where you breathe the noxious air and are constantly assailed by a nerve-scraping din that induces tension and adds weight to the emotional stresses of an urban environment. Or suppose you go to work for an asbestos factory. Or in a coal mine. Or, suppose you become a heavy drinker and smoker. Take drugs, abuse your body. Don't get proper rest. Or eat white bread and white sugar and sugary pies and cakes and other "junk" foods filled with additives and preservatives. You obviously are lopping years off of your life and you won't be able to count on your genes to overcome all the bad environmental and personal factors that go into making your life—and your life span.

There is no gene for longevity, as far as we know. There are only "bad" genes that can increase the probability of contracting or developing a fatal disease, of heightening your susceptibility to enemy agents that lurk in ambush to damage or destroy the human body.

Hippocrates, the father of medicine, noting individual susceptibility to disease, attributed these differences to variations in the blend of "humors." Today we refer to constitutional differences. The occurrence of many diseases in families points to a genetic basis for such constitutional differences.

For instance, heart attacks seem to occur in some families more frequently than in others. Narrow coronary arteries influence the incidence of heart attacks.

This could have a genetic basis, but also the size of the vessels can be influenced by physical activity.

Since there are no "good" genes for longevity, only "bad" ones with a negative influence, the doctors who studied the *viejos* for clues theorized that the isolated valley might represent an instance where "bad" genes simply didn't exist. And thus, they speculated that the genetic factor could be especially significant in the longevity of the Vilcabamba aged.

The Ecuadorian doctors, who had gone to the valley in 1969, promulgated the theory that Vilcabamba had been a "closed" community, with no mixing from the outside. They liked to say that these were "white" people—meaning descendants of Europeans, or non-Indian. But even if they were of European stock with Spanish forebears, the Spaniards were not all that "white," as they had been conquered by dark-skinned Moors before they invaded the New World. If the speculation were valid, it would support the theory that the *viejos'* longevity might have been attributable, to a large extent, to the fact that they had over the years bred out, as it were, any "bad" genes.

The legend propagated by the Quito doctors—based, obviously, on their speculation, only—went like this: A group of Spaniards, dating back to the fifteenth century conquests, and their descendants were barricaded behind the mountains, reproducing themselves, with apparently no infusion of other genetic strains from the outside.

When I got to the village, I had the same impression as Dr. Alberto Avila—the *viejos* appeared to be of European lineage. This came as a surprise because descendants of the Incas and earlier Indian tribes live throughout the Andes.

In the days when the eastern sector of South America—including modern-day Peru and Ecuador—comprised a vast empire ruled by the Incas, the indigenous Indians preferred living in the mountains. They built their centers of power and culture in Cuzco and Quito, cities that are twice as high as our mile-high city of Denver.

After the Conquest the Spaniards clearly demonstrated their preference for the coast, and thus through the remaining centuries the vast lonely stretches of the Andes were inhabited by the descendants of Incas, who continued to live in their traditional ways, with a different lifestyle and a different set of values from the white man of European stock. And they continued to speak the Quechua language, a native tongue that survived Spanish tutelage.

In the early 1960s, I had lived in Peru and I had visited many communities throughout the Andes where the purebred Indians still live. But in Vilcabamba, few look Indian. I was intrigued to find an isolated pocket of people who spoke Spanish, not Quechua, whose thought patterns stemmed from Unamuno and Santayana, not from tribal councils, and whose general appearance was more European than Indian in clothes, style and manner. I saw many *viejos* with blue and green eyes, and children and young adults who had blond hair and looked as much a product of western culture as I did.

Any visitor to the Sacred Valley of Ecuador might easily speculate that genetics play a significant role in the lives of the *viejos*. For instance, you might walk down the street in Vilcabamba and meet an old man and you hear his name is Carpio. You continue a few steps and meet another old man and you hear his name is Carpio. So, you might conjecture, both men are old and both are named Carpio. And you might wonder, are their genes therefore special?

Miguel Carpio was a special Old Man, no doubt about it. He lived next to the Churo *casa* where I frequently stayed, and to visit with Carpio I had to walk only ten or twenty steps. The simple house where Carpio lived with his large family had a front area used as a general merchandise store. Usually a son or a daughter was out front, minding the store.

They were elaborately courteous and courtly in manner. They always welcomed me like I was family, opened their arms to me, and insisted that I take a seat. And they offered me whatever food they might have. Their *casa* had little more furniture than a bare bench. Yet, their simple hospitality had a regal quality to it, as if they were commanding, "Come into my beautiful palace and rest on my velvet divan."

I asked Carpio if he thought that there was something about his family tree that had enabled him to live so long. He saw life not scientifically—genes to cells to complex organisms to species—but rather more philosophically. "But no," he said emphatically, "I do not believe that I have lived a long life because of a special family tree." Then he said quite simply, "It was my destiny." Medical authorities would despair of Carpio's metaphysical view of what sustained him. He told how he had fought in skirmishes against the Peruvians and a bullet had lodged in his stomach—and he showed me a long gash to prove his story. "That was the only time I ever needed a doctor. But it was not he who saved me." Then he restated his conviction: "A bullet cannot kill you, it is only destiny that determines when you die. *Lo que mata es el destino.*"

Unlike his daughters, Carpio loved to tell his age, or let's say, the age he believed himself to be. "My real age is 127 years. I have 12 sons, 98 grandsons, 70 great-grandsons and 72 great-great-grandsons." Carpio admitted frankly he had children outside wedlock: "I had women from the street." Then he added, "But I recognized my children, I gave them my name."

Old Erazo, on the other hand, confessed that he had sired children whom he had not recognized. The point is that there are thousands of Erazos, who for various reasons have had children they never saw or never recognized, and that it is difficult to determine our forebears and the importance of the genetic factor in our lives.

In Vilcabamba, however, no one could forget the genetic factor since the residents seemed to be one big family. For instance, the first time I mentioned to Carpio's daughter that I planned to go into the mountains to visit Erazo, she replied, "Oh, he is of our same family."

I asked how Erazo and Carpio were related.

"They are cousins," she said.

This was a statement I heard repeatedly. I suggested to Dr. Avila that there must be cases of cousins marrying cousins.

"I believe so," he replied.

"Is this bad for the population?"

"When an infant is born with a defect, he dies," Dr. Avila said. "The 'advanced' civilizations have a grand problem. For instance, in the United States an infant may be born with many defects and they keep him alive. There are special instruments to keep him alive, special institutions. So a child can be born without arms, legs, without a mind, but they use all their forces to keep him alive. But in Vilcabamba if such an infant should be born, he would die."

The Sacred Valley child who was weak or "unfit" had little chance to survive in an area where the arts of medicine were primitive or nonexistent. Or, if he did somehow survive birth, he passed through a natural crucible that insured an uncommon strength against the ravaging assaults of nature, disease and accident.

Dr. Avila emphasized that, "All the old people were born locally, so that what you refer to in the United States as the Miami Beach phenomenon, that is, an ingathering of the elderly, cannot account for the age distribution in Vilcabamba."

Then, he added, "You'll find Indian names are few."

Over the past two decades I have travelled widely in Spain, and have come to appreciate the fortitude of the Spaniards. And on my first encounter with a *viejo* such as Manuel Ramon, I had thought, *he is a Spaniard.*

I imagined that he embodied the fortitude, courage, brute strength of old *Conquistadores* who overcame every obstacle on their path to gold and glory. They ruthlessly slaughtered millions of Indians, and when they were not fighting Incas, they warred against one another. Violence had bred violence, until it had become a lifestyle.

My initial encounter with Ramon came after I had

gone by foot for many miles along rocky paths and up torturous mountainsides. Weary, I positioned myself at a spot where two footpaths converged. I did not go to the top of the mountain because I felt I would lose my way, or follow the wrong path and miss Ramon on his way down.

I relaxed, with my back against a granite stone, and had begun to doze lightly when I heard a stirring of leaves or sensed some movement on the path above me. I turned and saw this startling figure approaching. He had snow-white hair and white beard. He wore cotton pants and shirt, many patches visible at a glance, and a badly-frayed wool poncho. He looked like a man who had somehow survived a holocaust. Only Goya who in his last years painted ancient men could have captured the tenacity, the strength in Ramon's face. There was vigor etched in every line.

Over the weeks that followed after that first encounter, I gradually came to know him, and I asked Ramon to tell me about his forebears. I thought that since he had lived so long—he claimed 110—that he would tell me he had come from long-lived parents.

"No," he said, "my mother Ignacia Ramon died when she was thirty in an epidemic." This *peste* had also taken the life of his only sister, Rosa Ramon.

I asked about his father, but he confessed little knowledge of him. "I was born out of wedlock, *no era hijo de matrimonio*," he said. Ramon had no idea if his father lived to be a *viejo*. He had seen him only once, when he was a child. The father took him on an outing, to the nearby village of Celica, but Ramon had not liked being there, "and I came back home to my mother the next day."

One of the oldest of the *viejos*, Ramon, unfortunately, could shed no light on the longevity of his progenitors. Unlike modern scientists, he had no curiosity about the possibility that his history may have been preordained in his mother's womb.

As I came to know Ramon I saw that his physical characteristics that had appeared very Spanish were in some degrees misleading, for he was a breed apart

from the old *Conquistadores* who had been so ruth-
less in their war against the Incas.

Ramon possessed a gentleness, a compassion, a
quiet repose, a passivity, characteristics that we asso-
ciate with the Indian. While he had physical characteristics that no Indian has—such as his white beard—
he was surely a "child" of two cultures, the Spanish
and the Indian.

And this is what, in fact, Dr. Leaf and others in
the United States team learned about the *viejos*.

They had taken large vials of blood back with them,
to their laboratories at Massachusetts General Hospital
in Boston.

I had known that you can test blood by "type"—
that all of us are one type or another, "R" and "O" and
so forth.

But I did not know that group sampling of blood
can also indicate that one's heritage represents both
the Old and New World lineage. And this would hardly require doctors travelling 6,000 miles to determine.

The Spanish *conquistadores* came to the New World
without any of their wives or sweethearts, and they
had always from the very beginning married and
lived with Indian women, had children with them,
and given their children their names.

Moreover, as to the valley being "closed" to outside
immigration and marriages from other groups, this was
not likely the case.

While Vilcabamba seemed remote to those of us
who generally travel by automobile and jet, the descendants of the Incas and the old *conquistadores*—
Mestizos, as the people are called—had always travelled through the Andes, by horseback and by foot.
They knew the isolated, remote "hidden" valleys, even
if those of us from the modern world did not.

Dr. Leaf admitted that he learned little from the
group blood studies.

"I learned only enough to know what I would like to
know for a larger study," Dr. Leaf said. His statement
seemed to be indicative of all studies on longevity:
You learn one small answer and ten big questions.

"All that our blood studies have revealed thus far, is that the people are *mestizos*," Dr. Leaf said. "We can't say that the Old People are more inbred than anybody else. The technique we were using, blood groups, isn't specific enough. One could do it by genealogy, if you could track down family trees. And other specialists are now trying to do this."

The fact that the *viejos* are a mixture of Spanish and Indian races—and not "white" only, as the Quito doctors originally speculated—undoubtedly had increased their vigor.

The human race seems to need "new" blood. In Dr. Leaf's words, "we generally expect that too much interbreeding in one group produces a deterioration of the species."

The writer and gerontologist, Alex Comfort, has shown that children of genetically diverse members of a species are likely to be unusually vigorous and long-lived—so-called "hybrid vigor."

Dr. Leaf can't prove it by Vilcabamba studies, but he is convinced that heredity does play an important role. "I think people agree that there is something that goes in families, that heredity is a significant factor in long life," Dr. Leaf said.

Several studies of life expectancy of children of long-lived parents have indicated an advantage over that for children of short-lived parents. "The advantage, however, is a modest one," Dr. Leaf said. "One study of longevity based upon life insurance records, done by the researcher L. I. Dublin, indicated that children of long-lived parents had a life expectancy at age 20 that probably does not exceed three years the expectance of a similarly aged group whose parents were short-lived. This was the maximal statistical advantage that could be attributed to heredity according to this study."

Research on the influence of genetics and environment to longevity was done by F. J. Kallman and L. F. Jarvik. They did a long-term study of twins aged sixty years and over.

They studied both monozygotic (one egg) and dizygotic (two eggs) twins. Identical twins come from a single fertilized egg. They have the same complement of genes and their heredity is identical. Their studies showed that one-egg twins on the average die within five years of each other while the difference in age at death for two-egg twins is much larger.

The research, Dr. Leaf said, shows that in the case of identical twins, even when they were separated in different environments, "their life span turns out to be very similar."

He concludes that, "genetic factors do affect longevity."

However, it must be added, that these findings, as all such tests, were based on a mean or average.

In some cases of identical twins, their differences in age at death exceeded a decade.

Dr. Nathan W. Shock of Baltimore's Gerontological Research Center rated the genetic factor in longevity somewhat higher, pointing out that "studies have shown that children whose parents and grandparents reached the age of eighty and over lived an average three to six years longer than individuals whose parents died before reaching age sixty."

Our life expectancy has increased largely because of a reduction in infant mortality, as well as such environmental factors as sanitation, control of infectious diseases and improved nutrition. Dr. Leaf observed that, "Since few of us have the opportunity to choose our parents, it is fortunate that improving environmental factors have had such a favorable effect on health and longevity and still afford potential for further larger gains."

If longevity were mainly a matter of genetics, then there would be very little that we—or physicians— could do. On the other hand, if longevity is something that you can do for yourself—with the help of parents who give you a good start—then there are many new directions open to us.

My living among the *viejos* convinced me of one cardinal rule that all of us can remember: Living a long life is, in essence, a do-it-yourself proposition.

The *viejos* taught me, first and foremost, that you are your own best doctor. Put the genetic factor aside for a moment. Nobody is willed longevity. No pills, no artificial organs or glands, no magic medical wands can confer a reasonably healthy old age upon anyone. Only you can do this for yourself. Just remember that there is no one who knows your own body as well as you know it yourself.

The *viejos* have never thought, as some of us think, that a doctor can "cure" whatever malady comes along, because they have *never* seen doctors. (There has never been a doctor who lived in the village.) I never heard one *viejo* dwell on his aches and pains— and yet most old people you meet in this country will tell you about stiff joints, bad hearts, headaches. Many in the United States see doctors regularly and many become hypochondriacs. Having no doctors to visit, the *viejos* do not suffer this malady. They never exaggerate any illness or pain that they might have.

Even if you are now in your later years and are just awakening to the possibility of a do-it-yourself extension of life, there's plenty you can do that will show real results.

I came to see that the *viejos* of Vilcabamba lived long lives because they *earned* those extra years.

3

Exercise

The *viejos* of Vilcabamba have never been handicapped by the wheel as a mode of transport. They own no cars or bicycles. Nor do they have horses or burros to move them over the rugged landscape of the Sacred Valley. They simply walk. They walk to work and they walk home from work. That necessity enriches and strengthens them. The sedentary Americans say, "Let's take a walk," as if it were a challenge, a novelty, a course for which they deserve some unique credit. "Let's take a walk, it will be good for you"— this common exhortation would puzzle the *viejos*. For them, walking means getting from one point to another, no matter how distant. It is not a prescription for toning up the body, keeping the heart sound, the muscles alive. Yet their walking helps to keep them fit. They exemplify the old saying that each of us has two "doctors" —the left leg and the right leg. Sanchez and the other *viejos* literally lengthen their lives with their workday regimen on foot.

Walking, said President Eisenhower's heart specialist, Dr. Paul Dudley White, is the best exercise you can get. He urged us all to walk at least an hour every day. Or, he suggested, get a bicycle. Many of us remember when we walked to school, to church, to the store, to the post office, to the neighbors. Today, we drive to a drive-in cleaners, a drive-in theater, a drive-in bank and a drive-in restaurant. We drive to a golf course, and then ride in an electric-powered cart around the greens.

In the relatively short span of fifty years, the automobile has so altered our way of life that we seem oblivious to the small parodies it creates. Many of us drive to a park just to take a walk; we taxi to a "Y" to attend an exercise class. Walking sometimes seems almost disreputable, a profligate waste of time. The automobile is not just a mechanical replacement for the horse. To many Americans, the internal combustion engine has replaced the human feet. It represents an entirely new attitude, a new set of customs, and has ushered in an era of physical passivity. It determines the rhythm, the tempo, of our lives.

Once I followed Señor Ramon to his field of maize atop a mountain, and I wondered: How can he do it? He worked his field, with hoe or *lampa* and with a long sharp-bladed machete, moving about with a steady rhythm, a Rolex precision. The human body over millions of years has been fashioned to serve Señor Ramon and all the rest of us in strenuous, daily activities. We are designed to live as the *viejos* live, pushing ourselves to a physical limit.

Now with dramatic suddenness, we in our society have changed the pattern. First with the automobile. Then with television. A major part of our leisure time, formerly spent in outdoor walks or picnics, horseback riding, cycling, or camping expeditions or playing outdoor games now is spent in prone submission to a television set. Many of us spend entire days when our legs suffer from technological unemployment. The doctors who visited Vilcabamba were impressed, not so much by the fact that a few people had lived to the century mark or beyond, but because they were so physically active. They became convinced that exercise was one factor in longevity. They repeatedly said exercise could not be stressed too much in all of our lives.

Their comments make up a catalogue of sound advice:

Dr. Guillermo Vela of Quito:

> "The one bit of advice that I give my pa-
> tients is to take physical exercise. And the
> best exercise is walking. We all have this at
> our hand. We don't need to go to a club. It
> has been demonstrated 100 percent for 100
> percent that walking is the best exercise
> there is. But this is what we don't do. We go
> from the house to the car, from the car to the
> elevator.
>
> "I am impressed with the viejos' maintain-
> ing a high level of physical exercise for all of
> their lives. They get up early and they do not
> rest until the moment they go to sleep at
> night. They walk to get water, they straighten
> up around their house, they walk to a place to
> work—usually climbing up a mountain—and
> their activities involve miles and miles of
> walking."

Dr. Alberto Avila, also of Quito:

> "We doctors asked ourselves many times if
> we could do the work they do. As for myself
> I think that I could not do it; I personally
> could not." Then, turning to his own practice
> in Quito, the heart specialist continued: "I
> can speak from experience. Those with the
> greatest heart troubles are those who have
> the least physical exercise. They are execu-
> tives, they go each day to a desk.
>
> "The viejos, on the other hand, have never
> owned automobiles. They walk to the village,
> for church services and for any needed sup-
> plies. The fact that they never stop these
> long walks means they have less problems of
> the heart. This is a fact about their lives."

In this country, however, there have been studies
that show some rural people get *less* exercise than
many city people because men and women in the
country use a car to drive to their jobs and stores,

whereas many urban dwellers can, and frequently do, walk to work and to the stores.

Dr. Alexander Leaf of Boston:

> *"The old people all share a great deal of physical activity. The traditional farming and household practices demand heavy work, and male and female are all involved from early childhood to terminal days. Superimposed on the usual labor involved in farming is the mountainous terrain. Simply traversing the hills on foot during the day's activities sustains a high degree of cardiovascular fitness as well as general muscular tone."*

Dr. Leaf pointed to the case of José Maria Roa, 87, who makes adobe. "Forty years at the task have deformed his feet but increased the ability of his heart to fuel his body with oxygen. . . . Sedentary urbanites can do likewise with a sustained regimen of running, swimming, cycling."

Climbing mountains, running, swimming, cycling and jogging have one thing in common: they demand plenty of oxygen. One needs to push him or herself to a point of exhaustion to increase the maximum amount of oxygen that the body can process within a given time. The heart will then be in good condition to serve you, when you need to call on it, in an emergency. There is one way of staying flexible, and it is simple: Keep moving, don't stop, now or ever. We are told over again by medical experts, *use it or lose it*.

Once, I met Gabriel Sanchez trudging down from his field atop el Chaupi, and I asked him why he rose at dawn each day to make such an effort. "I would be ashamed, *seated* in the house all day," he said. On another occasion he told me that when he sat for too long a time, "I feel like dying." So each morning he got up, had his coffee and sweet potato, and started moving. Then he forgot his age, and any of his pains. All of his thoughts, all of his energy was devoted to the here and now, to the immediate challenge ahead of him. No long thoughts that would immobilize or discourage him. No idle reveries about the past that would cause his physical mechanism to wither from disuse.

All of the *viejos*, like Señor Sanchez, keep their motors running, as it were. Their pains are private matters to them, and they do not dwell on them. They keep moving, walking, working, as if in defiance of all the myths that age inhibits physical exertions. They sternly refuse to surrender to the debilitating concept of "being old." Instead, they remain doggedly flexible.

Doctors with increasing frequency are giving us results of tests showing that exercise pays off in longer and more healthy life spans. Here are a few examples:

—In Evans County, Georgia, Curtis Hames, M.D., reports the incidence of coronary heart disease higher among white male patients than among the county's black males, who are engaged in difficult manual labor, requiring a great degree of physical exertion.

A later study on a large segment of our adult population by J. C. Cassel confirms Dr. Hames's observation.

Cassel reports that two groups who engage in hard physical labor, white sharecroppers and black men, have less than half the incidence of heart disease as whites who are not engaged in that level of physical exertion.

Risk factors such as blood pressure, serum cholesterol level, smoking, body weight and diet could not account for the difference. The conclusion: It is the level of physical activity required by the blacks and white sharecroppers that largely protects them from coronary artery disease.

—A classic British study, done by J. N. Morris, compares the incidence of heart attacks among postal workers in London. Those who carry the mail bags and deliver the mail have a lower total incidence of heart attacks, less sickness and live longer than the workers who sit at desk jobs in the post office. The death rate among the workers who walk is one-third that of those who sit at their jobs.

This same study compares heart attacks among London bus drivers with those of bus conductors, who continually move around collecting fares. In this case, also, the physically active suffer fewer heart attacks and less illness than those with sedentary jobs.

—In the early 1960s, the town of Roseto in Pennsylvania boasted our country's lowest rate of cardiac deaths. J. I. Rodale visited Roseto in the summer of 1963 and wrote about it in the November, 1964, edition of *Prevention.*

He said that the first thing he noticed was the fact that there were so many steep, hilly streets in the town. Older Italians brought the habit of walking from their homeland. And he observed that walking up and down hills from childhood can be a big factor in one's good health. Walking increases the ability of the heart to operate more efficiently and generally reduces the blood pressure.

By the 1970s the so-called miracle town had become a typical American community—sick.

Why?

The diet had not changed all that much. (Although people formerly kept gardens, following the natural gardening techniques of their European forebears.)

The change from walking to driving undoubtedly plays a key role. As J. I. Rodale had pointed out, Roseto is built on a mountain slope and walking its steep streets is real exercise—the kind that strengthens the heart. And the kind that is easy to forego, when you've got four wheels at your doorstep. Driving is easier, but it does nothing for health.

The Rev. Gennaro Leone, pastor of Our Lady of Mt. Carmel, Roseto's Roman Catholic church, pointed to the exercise factor as the reason the citizens are not as healthy as they once were. "They drive cars," he said. *"Nobody walks anymore."*

Perhaps the most important benefit of exercise is its retarding effect on the process of arteriosclerosis, clogging of the arteries with fat. Muscular metabolism, especially that derived from the vigorous use of the leg muscles during walking, acts to prevent hardening and clogging of the arteries by a means not yet clearly understood.

Studies have been made of the Masai in Africa. Their feasts on meat raise their cholesterol levels to twice the limits recommended by the American Heart Association. Never having heard of the Heart Association, the Masai gulped tremendous amounts of cholesterol and obstinately refused to have heart attacks, thanks possibly to their penchant for exercise.

Exercise is not only good for the heart and mind, it is good for bones. Doctors tell us that all of us should in the course of our regular day be on our feet at least two hours. When we do not put weight on our bones they become susceptible to fracture.

The attention attracted by weightless existence in space flights made many aware of the fact that bones lose minerals when they are free of the stress of gravity, and that they gain the minerals back when they're once again subject to the pull and strain of carrying body weight.

But this is no new space-age discovery. Doctors have known for years that an immobilized limb will lose bone density, and regain its normal bone mineral content when the limb is put to use again.

Dr. Herbert A. DeVries, well-known for his successful work with the aging, says "It is an established fact that when a muscle is not at least occasionally stretched through its normal range of movement, it becomes shortened, often producing spasms and cramps which can be simply irritating or severely painful."

DeVries, professor of Physiology at the University of Southern California for many years, and also Director of the university's Mobile Laboratory for Physiology and Aging Research, states, "In animal experiments it has been shown that biochemical changes in the tissues which typically accompany aging also can be brought about by *immobilization*. These findings point to the importance of physical activity in the maintenance of normally functioning connective tissues."

Dr. Charles Bonner has written (in *Geriatrics*, June,

1969) about successful bone rehabilitation efforts at Cardinal Cushing Rehabilitation Center, Cambridge, Massachusetts. He learned that even the old bones of elderly patients, suffering from osteoporosis, or loss of bone density, and long bedridden, can be stimulated to new bone formation if a skilled, committed medical staff encourages and supervises appropriate mobilization and physical therapy.

A metabolically active skeleton has a constant turnover of minerals. Drs. Howard Rasmussen and Maurice Pechet, writing in *Scientific American* (October, 1970), report that the turnover of bone minerals "allows remodeling of the skeleton to enable it to deal with the developing mechanical stress of the body. It is as if each bone were an elaborate Gothic structure in which a resident engineer, in response to changes in stresses, continually directs the replacement of supporting arches with new ones providing a slightly different center of structural thrust."

The lesson we can derive from the *viejos* is plain: Each gives his or her bones a daily job to do, activating the "resident engineer" to perform its task of creating new bone formation.

Also, the *viejos* spend most of their waking hours out-of-doors. And Vilcabamba is blessed with an "eternal spring" of sunny days.

Much bone weakness in our country that used to be considered unavoidable in the elderly disappears when sunshine is added to the diet.

Research in Great Britain reveals a significant proportion of hip fractures in the elderly may not be due to osteoporosis, a gradually developing and difficult-to-cure disorder. Rather, they can be the result of a temporary condition—deficiency in vitamin D.

Dr. J. E. Aaron and colleagues report in *The Lancet* (February 16, 1974) that lack of outdoor sunshine is perhaps the major reason many older people develop vitamin D deficiency. Throughout history, sunshine—not food—has been the major source of vitamin D for the human species. The ultraviolet rays of the sun convert lipids, a key component of living cells in the skin, into the same vitamin D that you and I get when we take a fish liver oil supplement.

Getting outdoor sunshine regularly—as well as exercise—remain vital health measures—and they are not overlooked by the remarkable *viejos,* who seemingly never suffer fractures.

U.S. doctors said the lives of the *viejos* brought home to them the threat that the sedentary occupations and sedentary recreations make against our lives. The more sedentary our lifestyle, the more dangerous it is.

Many are recognizing this. Every day in Washington, D.C., I see officeworkers leave their sedentary jobs at midday and instead of going out to lunch, they jog across Memorial bridge, or through Rock Creek park. The Pentagon has become a beehive of high-ranking joggers.

Increasingly, Americans are turning to physical exercise to escape illnesses, fatigue and early deaths. A survey made in 1974 for the President's Council on Physical Fitness and Sports revealed that 55 percent of the U.S. adult population—some 60 million people—participate in exercises, such as hiking, jogging, skiing, bicycling, tennis, karate and yoga. We are learning that the human body runs down faster than an automobile when it is just left idle, without ever running the motor.

The *viejos* develop their bodies and keep them toned and supple simply because they constantly use them. One striking sample was Manuel Pardo. Señor Pardo was ninety-six and he still did day labor at *hacienda* Palmira, a distance of ten miles. Sometimes he went there by autobus, but oftentimes he would walk.

And what was the best thing in life? I asked him.

"To work, *trabajar,* there is no other thing. To fight, *luchar,* for the life."

I was surprised to hear Señor Pardo say "work" rather than *amor* was the best in life. I asked him about this, and he replied that we can't live without love. But rather than a man's love for a woman he spoke of

a love for own's own life, *su propia vida.* He explained
it this way: "I work for a patron. But I also work for
myself, *mi dignidad.* It has to be good work."

Had his life been full? I asked.

"Yes, God has helped me. I've had a life with little
sickness. I've worked with the *barreta, lampa, hacha*
—eight and ten hours a day."

When I wanted to visit with Señor Pardo, I would
walk in a circle around the central plaza and often we
would chance to meet each other.

Once by way of greeting I said: "What a beautiful
day."

"It will rain," he told me.

We talked of going to visit his sister Sara and her
husband Alberto Roa. Would it rain?

He and I started out from the square, but then it began to rain and we returned to the village and sat on a
bench in front of Carpio's.

Then he said "*Vamonos,*" let's go, rain or no rain.

We began the hike up a steep incline, past the *hacienda* Casa Blanca. The path was steep and muddy.

"We'll go little by little, *poco a poco,*" he said.

But I could hardly keep up with him, *poco a poco.* I
wondered what it would be like if he were in a rush.

Watching his steady, determined march forward, I
reflected: He teaches me; only he can show me, only
he who has been over the route. He can give an example of how to live all your days. He *walks* his words.
(Walking, said one gerontologist, is the closest thing to
an anti-aging pill now available.)

I felt relaxed, happy, contented, buoyed with a
childlike élan. Doctors cannot yet explain in physiological terms why exercising the body produces a sense of
relaxation. But we know that we can break the vicious
cycle of muscular disuse and muscular tension by simply taking a walk.

Señor Pardo and I crossed a rope-and-steel suspended bridge, made by hand, and he showed me how
to place my feet so I wouldn't fall. It was such an effort
to get up the mountain; it was hot, it was steep, it was
struggle. All along the way I kept repeating to my-

self, *life is struggle*, it is the constant effort of putting one foot in front of the next.

Gerontologists now are attempting to learn what keeps an eighty-year-old man with as good a heart-beat as a fifty-year-old man. As one doctor said: "He must be different."

Hiking with Pardo, I found it difficult to believe I was forced to make such a determined effort to keep up with a near centenarian.

"We can rest at the *casa*," he urged me on. "It isn't far now."

I was pushing myself as fast as I could move, through mud, up an almost perpendicular incline. Starting out, I had felt like a little child; now, approaching exhaustion, I felt older than he. My body and mind felt permeated by a craving to rest, to collapse on the spot, as the precipice grew steeper, more difficult to climb.

"You walk better than I do," I said.

"*It is necessary to suffer a little*," he told me. Keep going, push yourself. Don't be too soft, too easy on yourself.

My muscles ached in a way as to mock Pardo's encouraging words. What does he know, this ancient freak, this oddity of the mountain valley? What does he prove except that he had trained himself to humiliate younger visitors? These unfair and ungracious thoughts came from my hurting muscles. I insisted on talking, perhaps only to slow Pardo down and thereby to give myself a rest.

I asked him, Did he like to ride horses?

"No, I prefer to walk. By foot, *a pie*, you can go anywhere—places where a horse or mule can't go." And he moved on, without pausing.

Pardo apparently did not have time for ailments. I thought of how so many of our old people spend their time, seated, dwelling on their infirmities. One suffers with muscular stiffness, another has arthritis, and the list of old folks' ailments seems endless: impoverished, degenerative organs, ill-defined discomfort and the tendency to tire quickly. But Manuel Pardo seemed to be that rare exception to what happened to *other* old men. He was way out front, coaxing me on, assisting me across difficult hurdles, holding fence wires up for me to crawl under. He seemed well oiled in all his joints. And in terms of our "fatigability," I was the ninety-six-year-old and he was half my age.

Once we were at the top, we were greeted by Sara and Alberto and because I was bone weary, not to mention slightly depleted in spirit, from the struggle, the opportunity to rest on a wooden bench outside their mud hut was like a well-earned trophy. As I sat resting I gazed at the peaceful valley below, and it had never seemed more beautiful. Walking had somehow made me appreciate it all the more.

After 2,000 years, a long series of medical studies here and abroad, embodied in the lives of Gabriel Sanchez, Manuel Ramon, Manuel Pardo and other *viejos* of Vilcabamba, affirm the words of Hippocrates: regular exercise, especially walking, is a person's best "medicine." Hippocrates prescribed brisk walks, short walks, early morning walks, after-dinner walks, night walks. Early morning walks were for emotional disturbances. Brisk walks were to reduce weight and keep one's figure trim. The Greek writer Pliny the Elder described walking as one of the "Medicines of the Will" . . . and it still is. You have to have willpower to get out of bed and climb a mountain and work all day.

The *viejos* of Vilcabamba—as did our parents or grandparents—took exercise routinely in their lives. Walking five or ten miles, working hard on a farm all day, going into the woods, cutting down trees, this was accepted as routine. In one or two generations, what was once routine has become outmoded, a target of jest and ridicule, an eccentric habit. A man or woman who insisted on walking a dozen miles to and from work today—at least in the United States—would be regarded as weird.

Once, at a restaurant, I overheard women at a table chatting. One commented, "My sister is visiting me from Lithuania, and she says what surprises her most about this country is that, as she puts it, '*I never see anyone walking.*'"

Her remark brought to mind visits I have made to Holland, Belgium, Yugoslavia, France and Germany, and how I had marvelled at seeing so many beautiful old couples out walking. They walk through the public gardens, they walk to the country, they walk up mountains, they walk to the opera, they walk miles, perhaps all morning, to get to a favorite restaurant, or they walk all afternoon to get to their favorite wine *stube*. Walking for them is a way of life.

They believe walking is the simplest, the most inexpensive and the best exercise. Many healthy Europeans will tell you they do not believe in diets. Rather than dieting, they will urge you to take a walk.

In the United States, walking went out of style to the point that people began writing books about it as if they had discovered a strange phenomenon, reminding one and all that we *can* walk and that it will be good for us.

In her book, *The Right Way to Walk for Health*, Mary Jo Takach tells us that a brisk walk can keep you in a good physique, eliminate fatigue, prevent and cure heart disease, and if you suffer with arthritis, it will ease your pain.

Aaron Sussman and Ruth Goode in *The Magic of Walking* tell us, "Walking is not only the nondieting diet . . . it is the prescription without medicine, the cosmetic . . . that is sold in no drugstore. It is the tranquilizer without a pill, the therapy without a psychoanalyst, the fountain of youth that is no legend."

Some people worry that exercising will increase their appetite and they will eat more and get fatter. In Vilcabamba, I found I ate more food than normally, but that I actually lost weight. I attribute it to the walking I did.

A study conducted at the University of California at Irvine, under the direction of Dr. Grant Gwinup (reported in May, 1975, issue of *Internal Medicine*, publication of the American Medical Association) would bear this out.

It showed that obese persons lost plenty of weight by exercise alone, without any dietary change. Dr. Gwinup said that brisk walks, beyond a half hour a day, and preferably two to three hours, are the best form of exercise for taking off excess poundage.

Exercise not only is good for your figure, but also calms the mind and enables us to entertain our best thoughts. Beethoven composed while strolling every morning. Mozart said his favorite time to compose was while walking after a meal. Robert Burns often composed poetry when "holding the plow." Pasteur walked the corridors at the Ecole Normale, "meditating the details of his work."

The very act of walking somehow clears the cobwebs out of your mind and gives you a fresh perspective. "Walking," said Rousseau, "has something which animates and vivifies my ideas."

But, one might say, I have never exercised—and it's too late to start now.

Doctors, however, say that it is never too late for most of us to build back the muscles we have lost with our sedentary years. "Long range studies," Dr. Nathan W. Shock said, "reveal that 70- and 80-year-old persons can be put on an exercise program that builds up their muscles in the way that you can build up a 20-year-old."

Dr. Herbert A. DeVries, physiologist at the University of Southern California, made many tests proving that older people can recapture at least part of their youthful energy with special exercise programs. He found that a vigorous six-week regimen of toe touching, jogging and swimming for one hour, three times a week, transformed a volunteer group of more than 100 men ranging in age from 52 to 87. Their heart and lungs functioned better, the flow of oxygen through the body improved and blood pressure dropped. The men reported that they were able to work longer and better, and that their sex lives had improved. Most encouraging of all for nonathletes, the improvement seemed to have little connection with how athletic a man had been in his youth.

Thus, it's never too late to start a regular exercise program to build up your muscles. I myself hope to remember Pardo's advice: *you have to suffer a little.* But keep going. I know if I want to stay in as good a shape as Pardo, I will walk at least an hour every day. Briskly. And, when possible, up and down some hills.

4

Environment

More than 2,000 years ago the Greeks recognized the importance of the emotional and psychological links to one's environment.

Hippocrates states that the physical and mental characteristics of the various populations of Europe and Asia are determined by the topography of the land, the quality of the air and the water, and the abundance and nature of the food.

These natural factors had shaped the lives of the *viejos*, influenced their outlook and attitudes as much as their encounter with the human family.

And in my own case, I know that having been born on the plains of Texas, where I saw space as beauty, the topography of the land and other regional influences helped shape my life.

Today in my urban existence I cannot measure the loss of beauty in my life as I shut myself off, in a high-rise apartment, from grass and trees, brooks and springs, and clean air.

I knew, packing my bags in my Washington, D.C. apartment, that I would be leaving one "world" with its polluted skies for another "world" in South America, a world free of belching industrial chimneys, aerosol sprays, automobile exhaust—a world with its own brand of hardships and rigors imposed, not by man's drive to progress, but by nature.

To reach the Andean village, I flew first to Quito, the Ecuadorian capital 3,000 miles due south of New York. As my plane dipped over the city, the gigantic Andes provided a backdrop that was at once breath-catching and awesome. In these mountains the mighty Amazon begins as a network of trickling streams. Impenetrable rain forests challenge any but the most hardy adventurer. These natural wonders eclipse the handiwork of man, the cathedrals, citadels, monuments and mausoleums.

My heart seemed to quicken when the pilot said, "Look below—there is where the equator crosses a glacier on the 18,996-foot Cayambe volcano." And there was Quito, only fourteen miles south of the equator but nearly two miles above sea level, and a sparkling gem stuck on a mountain plain. From the air, Quito can be said to resemble a necklace of diamonds and sapphires glinting around the lower slopes of the volcano Pichincha. This 9,350-foot-high city, once the home of the famous Inca god-emperor Atahualpa, has survived volcanic eruption, earthquake—and conquest by Inca and Spaniard. Only two other pre-Columbian capitals in the Western Hemisphere—the Aztec capital of Mexico City and Cuzco, the first Inca capital—are as old as Quito.

After a rest in Quito, where a winter coat felt good, I bought a bus ticket and proceeded south towards Vilcabamba. The antiquated bus, "made in Ecuador" from junk parts of every vintage and model vehicle since year one of the automotive industry, was loaded, with every inch of sitting and standing space taken. Bundles of hay, bicycles and baggage were piled on top and insecurely fastened by rope and belts.

The bus careened up and down along "the Avenue of the Volcanoes," passing Cotopaxi that towers 19,347 feet and is one of the world's highest active volcanoes. A few miles outside of Quito, it began to rain. For twelve hours, without moving from the bus—there were no "rest stops" as such—I felt melded into the crowded bus, pressed so closely to others I did not know where I left off and they began. I felt a small part of a seething whole, a cellular addition to a multiplying mass embarked upon an adventure in growth and learning.

An overnight stop in the beautiful city of Cuenca, with its Spanish-styled, pastel-colored stucco buildings, gave me a chance to stretch and recover my identity. Then, back on a bus for another long journey through the towering mountains.

Second only to the Himalayas in height, the Andes slice Ecuador into three separate "worlds": a steamy jungle to the east, an arid desert along the coast, and the mountains in between. When the Spaniards came, searching for gold, they marched from the desert into the soaring peaks of the Andes. They braved frigid winds and confronted terrifying gorges and glacier-mantled peaks whose icy snow the fierce equatorial sun never melts. They reached the summit of a peak expecting to find themselves on the top of the world, only to look out upon other peaks, all alive with furious torrents and hideous chasms whose depths they feared and could not fathom.

Geologically, the Andes are still new, still changing and still subject to every possible catastrophe such as earth tremors and landslides. Besides three main chains of mountains that run north-south, there are lesser ranges that weave in and out of these *cordilleras* like a jigsaw at work, creating pockets of small and large valleys and walling their inhabitants off from one another.

To understand why a village such as Vilcabamba could have been "lost" in time for hundreds of years, one must visualize these isolated pockets as a natural maze without connecting channels, except those eventually carved by brave pioneers. One of the *conquistadores*, Orellana, marched south from Quito—crossed the splintered porphyry and granite Andean slopes and descended into the lush tropical jungle. Starving, he boiled the soles of his shoes, and having eaten them, sailed down a river in search of food. He kept sailing—for 4,000 miles, across the earth's midriff, having inadvertently "discovered" the Amazon.

Two hundred years later the French savant La Condamine and the Prussian scholar Humboldt arrived in Ecuador. Humboldt wrote about the rocks, the geological nature of the deposits, the volcanic phenomena, aspects of the *cordillera*, the marvels of the vegetation, the beauty of the mountains, the magnificence of the rivers. He was among the first to draw attention to the ethnological relationship between the Mongolians and the New World aborigines.

But generally the mountains and valleys of Ecuador were undisturbed by alien intruders, silent and unknown to the outside world. We know little, for instance, about the medicinal herbs that the residents say protect them from such maladies as cancer and heart disease. No one has made serious, long-range studies of the soil contents, although many have commented on the fecundity of the plant life in the Sacred Valley. The world beyond the Valley has benefited from one miracle drug, first discovered in the Valley. This was quinine, a bark the Spaniards named *cinchona* because it saved the life of the Condesa de Chinchon when she suffered with malaria in 1638.

Few serious scholars and explorers have gone into the area since the days of the *conquistadores* and La Condamine and Humboldt. Even today, Ecuadorians in Quito do not travel to the long-isolated southern province of Loja, the state in which Vilcabamba is located. Being on the other side of the mountains in Ecuador is like being on the other side of the moon. Travel is laborious and slow, even today. It takes two days by air to get from Quito to Loja—with an overnight stop that one must make in Guayaquil. In road miles, the trip from Quito to Loja is only 350 miles, but I sat on a bus for 30 hours to cover that distance. Often, because of landslides and washed-out roads, the trip can take a week.

In Loja, a province capital which still has a frontier atmosphere with horse-drawn carts in the main thorōughfares, I rested overnight. And the next morning I boarded another antiquated bus for the last lap of my journey to Vilcabamba.

The bus pulled out of Loja, at an altitude of 7,200 feet, and wound its way over a narrow, twisting dirt road up to 11,000 feet. Along the way, small clusters of workmen alternately were repairing and widening the road, preparing for the tourists that Loja officials hope to attract to the area.

After three hours of slowly chugging up and briskly coasting down the mountain road, inching our way past landslides, the bus turned a corner and far in the distance one could see the Sacred Valley with its church and cluster of houses. It seemed that God and man working with the same instruments and purpose had created this scene. It was all so harmoniously arranged that it appeared to have been executed on a canvas and set in a frame.

There was an aspect of otherworldliness, a sense of discovery, so pristine that one imagined he had caught the Creator in the midst of His handiwork. It evoked images of faraway places, one's dreams of Tibet, or Persia or ancient Peking. It was like viewing a misty pastoral scene on an old Chinese scroll: the beauty was suggested more than it was explicitly delineated. One's mind conjured up scenes from Pearl Buck's *The Good Earth,* for in this Andean hinterland, as in countless villages in China and around the world, the cycle was the same: life and death and new life, all allied to the "good earth." As on a long and tranquil ocean voyage time seemed almost suspended. The stillness suggested that the valley might have been entombed for a millennium.

The village, nestling at 4,500 feet among mountains covered with lush tropical foliage, was untouched by neons, mercantile bustle and those smoking portents of a polluted environment. It reminded one at a glance of the mythical "Shangri-La" of James Hilton's *Lost Horizon.*

As we neared the valley, it appeared like a picture

postcard suddenly animated, with the village and its
church steeple arranged by the photographer for maximum effect.

We crossed a rickety bridge over the Chamba river,
one of two rocky streams that flow through the village,
providing it with an ample water supply. Native wom-
en in brightly colored dresses were seated along the
riverbank, washing clothes and gossiping in the noon-
time sun.

Seeing the women by the stream, and *viejos* working in distant fields, I thought they seemed to fit into
the texture of the Sacred Valley as naturally as animals
in the forest. Like the springs, streams, hills, rocks and
vegetation—like the sun and sky itself—the people in
the valley radiate a sense of belonging. They seem a
part of the tranquility and continuity of the earth that
one remembers from his or her childhood in the
woods and mountains.

I was inescapably assailed, upon seeing the valley
for the first time, by the feeling that *This was once my
home, This is where I began. Only the viejos have not
been uprooted. Only they had the wit to stay home.* I
realized that those who stay rooted are geographically
stable, an organic unit of sprawling landscape. They
represent the persistence of its character, its beauty. I
know that my forebears had their earliest homes in
such pastoral settings, and such memories prompted
the atavistic thought that I had discovered a horizon
lost somewhere in my unrecollected past.

The bus, with much blaring of horns, came to an
abrupt stop on the east side of the Vilcabamba central
plaza. I got off, and with bag in hand walked across a
dirt street to a two-story building and entered a general merchandise store. I walked past bags of rice and
bags of beans and bolts of material, and came to the
owner, Manuel Churo. After only a few words, he let
me know we were two kindred spirits, since he,
too, had come from the "outside world." He was a native of Quito, and he seemed to welcome another
stranger. He introduced me to his señora, Rosa Cabre-
ro Churo, and when I asked where I might stay in the

village they agreed to rent me a room above their general store.

It had no conveniences, no visible or invisible links to Hilton or Sheraton. It was simply a place to sleep. I was glad to take it, and I arranged to pay for it by the week, a payment that would not have taken care of my tips for a day at the Waldorf. I reached this treasured abode in the Churos' loft by walking up a flight of outside stairs. The room had no furniture except a single frame bed and a small child's bedpan on which I had to carefully arrange myself to make sure I hit the pot and not the floor.

I immediately learned that I had nothing to turn on, nothing to turn off. There was no electricity (there was a town generator but the motor was broken). So when there was light it was from a kerosene lamp, or, in my case, I had a small candle, but I would not use it much. When it got dark, I would yield to the village custom and go to bed. The people in the village have no TV and only a few battery-operated radios. There are no newspapers or magazines, and little communication. To contact Loja, one goes to a two-room hut and asks for a "conference" and the operator, Gonzalo Bastidas, arranges for you to talk on the one phone.

I had no mirror, no water with which to brush my teeth. I was truly liberated from the time-consuming feminine activities such as shaving my legs and under my armpits, spraying deodorant under my arms, and plucking my eyebrows, painting my nails, curling my hair.

Living in the Sacred Valley was like being a child again. I waked each morning at sunrise, brushed my hair into a ponytail, slipped on my every-day-of-the-week clothes, and I was ready to greet the day, the Vilcabamba way. At five o'clock each morning, life seemed to burst open right below my window. My alarm was not with the loud clanging of church bells, as one so frequently hears in Latin American *pueblos*, but rather the roaring of a motor and the honking of a loud horn that signaled the imminent departure of the first autobus for the provincial capital of Loja.

The first morning I jumped into a skirt and sweater and went out looking for coffee. Few in the village seemed to be stirring yet. I asked the bus driver where he had his coffee, and he told me that he would wait until he got to Loja, and I imagined he could have added, "I will wait for that other world, that world in which I can walk into a real restaurant, and there will be tables and tablecloths and menus and waiters to serve me, and there will be plenty of food, and I can order whatever I wish to eat."

I watched passengers board the bus, and I, too, wanted to go. I felt that I desperately wanted to escape, and I knew a near panic at being left behind, in what seemed then to be a village of nothingness.

In my first stroll around the central square, I saw that the church dominated the small village. It was not especially impressive or even large, but it nevertheless dwarfed the other structures.

Small adobe *casas* radiated from the square along narrow, dirt streets. The houses, a few with tile but most with thatched roofs, had dirt floors, and were not homes in our sense of the word so much as shelters for the night.

If you go alone to a strange village there is the danger of being "taken in"—and in Vilcabamba, I was "taken in" but by people who were kindhearted and who, having been lonely, could imagine that I, too, might be lonely.

Since I am by nature as friendly as a stray pup, I began to brush up against people, to talk with them, and to relate, one to one, with them. I have always found that if one communicates to a *latino* the simple message, "I want to be your friend," he is worthy of the trust.

And within a few days, I began to make friends, and one, a Señor Toledo, lived in the village but also had a farm, *huerta*, outside the village where he kept a horse. I told him that I wanted to borrow the horse to ride out into the mountains to visit the *viejos*, who worked *huertas* high in the *sierra*. And Señor Toledo agreed to bring his *caballo* into the village for my use.

Early the next morning I put on my slacks, a blouse and sweater and shoes, and went downstairs to find Señor Toledo, standing by a spavined mare that in her world looked as ancient as any of the centenarians. Señor and Señora Churo and the police lieutenant with a long impressive name, Teniente Politico Celso Flavio Benitez Suarez, and a few others had gathered to watch my leaving, my *despedida*.

Remembering from my Texas training how to mount a horse, I put my left foot in the left stirrup and with, I hoped, some insouciance pulled myself *up*. But as I went flying *up*, the old remnant of an English saddle came tumbling *down*, so that instead of finding myself triumphantly aboard the horse, I found myself on my backside, sitting in the dirt. No one laughed, however. And Señor Toledo busily rearranged the saddle and tightened the girth. The police lieutenant said I needed a *sombrero*, and one of the onlookers, a centenarian named Señora Toledo, and a distant relative of the owner of the horse, took off her small straw hat, and handed it to me. It would not go *on* my head, but rather merely perched there. But I thanked her, and kicked my knees into the belly bones of the mare, and we took off at a trot.

I felt slightly apprehensive but excited about what lay ahead. Along a route roughly described to me, I kept asking, "Where is el Chaupi?" "*¿Donde está* el Chaupi?" A foreigner or *gringa* astride a horse was not the most common sight in the elevated backwaters of Ecuador, but the few people I encountered were friendly, gracious and accommodating.

As I kept on the path to el Chaupi, the mountain where Sanchez worked, I tried to imagine how anyone, of any age, would have the strength to climb the peaks that rimmed this peaceful valley. I was impressed by the tranquility, the slowed-down pace of life. I passed flowering *arupo* that reminded me of cherry blossoms.

The narrow dirt road took me through lush untended foliage, and thick green fields of sugar cane, corn, bananas, tobacco. I soon shed the sweater over my blouse, tying the sweater around my waist. As the horse and I jigged and jogged along, the ancient English saddle promising me no relief from future sores, I felt blessed by the typical Vilcabamba weather, bright, temperate, dry. The sky and air were all promise. The day being so special made me feel a special person, my spirit became as expansive as the world was wide. I saw beauty all around me.

Although only four degrees south of the equator, Vilcabamba, because of its altitude, never suffers with the relentless equatorial heat. It enjoys a fairly steady 68° F. temperature, reminding me of the weather in certain regions of Colorado and New Mexico, especially Taos and Santa Fe.

Coming to the San Pedro river, I dismounted and while the horse grazed along the banks, I attempted to gauge the depth and swiftness of the stream. Momentarily I thought of our being swept downstream, and drowning. I do not fear death, but it is still an impenetrable mystery not amenable to rational argument.

After a rest along the river bank, I remounted the horse and coaxed him into the stream. He swam across without incident, carrying me to the other shore. We continued along a rugged path, leading upward, ever more steep. Eventually, I tied the horse to a gate and walked a steep incline to Sanchez' place, where I saw an old woman whose years and hardships had bent her almost double. She turned out to be Sanchez' second wife, Maria Petrona Yunga, and she told me she was ninety. I noted how her head hung over her chest, almost to her waist. Once her body must have been strong and straight as the eucalyptus, but now that body had shrunken to the size of a child of ten. Like any aged person, in any economic and social strata, in any part of the world, Maria Petrona Yunga had grown up, then she had grown down. Her husband, she said, was at the top of el Chaupi.

I determined to continue my climb up the mountain, in search of Sanchez. Maria Petrona Yunga stood beside me, our eyes squinting into the sunlight. "There he is," and she pointed out what to her trained eyes was a speck on the sky-high terraces. I knew Sanchez was there, because she had said he was, but just as I had puzzled over line drawings to "see" a cow in a barn so I puzzled over discerning a man's figure in the vastness of the green landscape, but without success. I knew the direction to follow, however —*up*.

I left the Sanchez *casa* and continued the trek up the mountain, following a trail the horse could ascend, but this trail became a ribbon of sharp rocks, so steep that I walked, and often even crawled ahead, leading the horse by the reins.

Eventually I reached the top, and there in his rocky field of maize I saw old Sanchez, who looked as I imagined the long-suffering Job "being old and full of days" might have looked, had he been able to step out of the pages of the Old Testament.

He was about five feet, five inches tall. He had an enormous chest that I assumed had developed during his decades of climbing into high altitudes.

He was in clean rags and sandals, leaning on his hoe, or *lampa*. He seemed a part of the mountain, another rock, as much an ingredient of the soil as its mineral contents. Indeed, he seemed to have stood there so eternally that he was now a monument to the theory held by many, among them the writer Lawrence Durrell, that landscapes so profoundly affect human development that human beings are expressions of their landscapes rather than their genes.

Sanchez obviously was surprised to see me, a stranger who had suddenly loomed before him, in his faraway mountain retreat where his only companions had been the insects and a few birds.

On my arrival at the mountaintop retreat, I had i
mediately sat down, exhausted. But this remarkal
viejo stood, his hands on the top of his hoe. Finally,
my insistence, he sat beside me. As we talked, I fou
him open to my gestures. We were being natura
tender and understanding with each other. He w
outgoing and candid, telling me of the saddest aspe
of his life, the loss of a son. The boy had gone to he
some Spaniards in distress, across the river, and t'
stream had been too swift, and the boy was caught
the currents, and drowned. His eyes were pools
grief as he relived that story, and it was plain that l
still carried the burden of the loss, endlessly wonde
ing why, why? The story of that dead son seemed
have welled up from a secret part of him, long burie
I wanted to attempt to get all the "facts" of the stor
but I sat knowing that I never could. I could, ho
ever, know "the truth" of his grief, his suffering.

Life, he seemed to say, was a mystery, and the my
tery was constantly before him, in his mind, in h
eyes. He had lived all of his life close to the grea
mysteries. Unlike modern man, he had never know
an office, never been barricaded behind walled rooms

Sanchez' life seemed to exemplify how environme
tal conditions can shape a man. We in our urban exi
tence cannot measure the loss of beauty in our lives a
we become "cave dwellers" in high-rise apartment
and offices.

Aristotle tried to imagine how men who had spen
all their lives under luxurious conditions in cave
would respond when given for the first time th
chance to behold sky, clouds, and seas. Surely, he ob
served, "These men would think that gods exist an
that all the marvels of the world are their handi
crafts."

D. H. Lawrence said that topography, geology an
climate give to each country "its own flowers, tha
shine especially there," and even more its own skie
which determine the moods of the people and the
landscape. I cannot visualize a Gabriel Sanchez, na

LOS VIEJOS —
"The Old Ones"

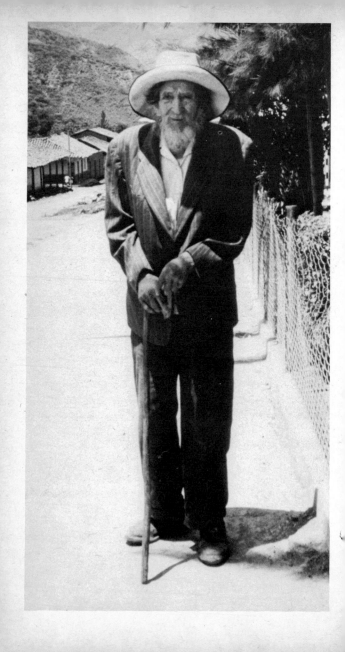

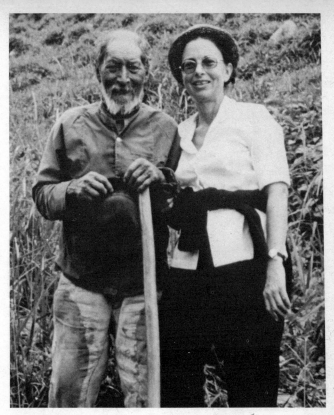

Gabriel Sanchez, who says matter-of-factly, "I am 113,"
continues to climb the steep el Chaupi mountain and work all
day with his crude hoe or *lampa*, cultivating a small plot
of corn. He called author Grace Halsell, here with him, little
doctor, *"doctorita."* She noted the patches on his clothes, the
poverty of his life. Yet, she admired his discipline, his philosophy.
His great age, she wrote, "made me feel my life had just begun!"

Opposite: When U.S. medical experts flew to Vilcabamba
they questioned Miguel Carpio, and other *viejos* about their diet
and exercise and hereditary background, but Carpio, 127,
said he lived a long and full life because "it was my destiny."
He once fought in a skirmish between Peruvians and Ecuadorians
and was hit by a bullet, but it didn't kill him because, again,
he believed it was fate that permitted him to live.

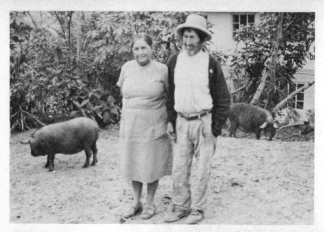

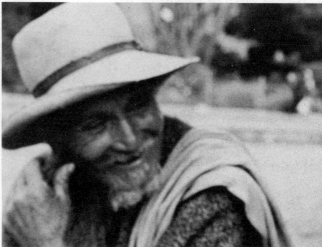

Top, left: Damian Lanche, 100, shown with one of his five children, Victoria, 65, lives in the nearby village of San Pedro, where he raises pigs. He gets up at 6 A.M. and takes no siesta — although he sometimes is in bed by 6 P.M. He does not smoke or drink hard liquor, but enjoys three cups of coffee a day.

Top, right: Right away, Micaela Quezada, 104, will tell you she's a virgin. She boasts about it, as some women might boast of having a Ph.D. Still, others in the village like to joke that one

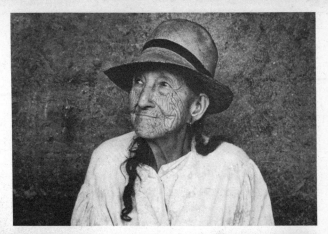

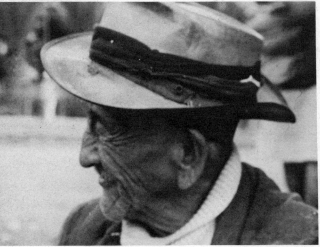

day she might get married to a widower, such as Carpio or Erazo. Not being caught up watching TV, the *viejos* talk often of romance, and they like to predict future marriages.

Bottom: Manuel Ramon, 110, left, enjoys a laugh with Gabriel Erazo, 132, right. The *viejos* build their lives around hard work, simple food and love. They are never too old to talk about romance, and they keep it alive in their lives. Also, they enjoy puns and laughter — and never take themselves too seriously.

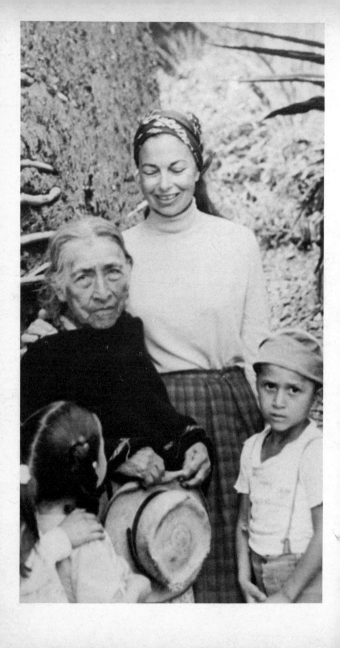

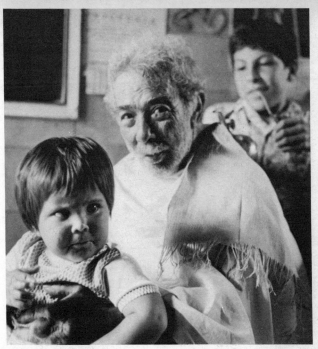

Angel Modesto, 91, and his great-grandson, Luis Fernando, not yet two, seem made for each other. The child is always playing near the old man or sitting in his lap — even when Modesto went to the one-chair barber shop to get his hair trimmed by a very young barber. In Vilcabamba anyone can cut hair, but sitting in the barber's chair makes it an important event.

Opposite: Senora Rosa Pizon, center, 93, is one of the few widows in the village without a family to look after her. Here she is shown with Grace Halsell and some of the Vilcabamba boys and girls who affectionately call Senora Pizon "grandmother."

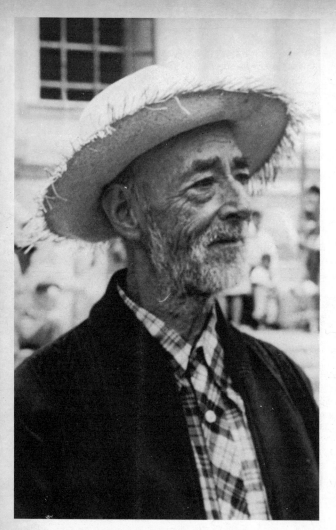

Celso Leon, 105, regularly attends services in the
Catholic church. The *viejos* are all religious and yet they
see life clearly, believing that the purpose of life is to learn
how to die. Senor Leon is an example of a simple, God-
fearing man who believes that what is required of man is to
"love mercy, do justice—and walk humbly before God."

tive of New York City, or a Gabriel Sanchez, who grew up in Chicago. He is of the soil, an organic part of the valley, immovable. He seemed an expression of his environment rather than of his genes.

Tolstoy, Chekhov and Dostoevski were formed to a degree by the vastness of their "mother" Russia just as a man from the plains of Kansas can be quite different from one born in an asphalt jungle ghetto of Watts or Harlem. James Baldwin wrote, "It means something to live where one sees space and sky or to live where one sees nothing but rubble or nothing but high buildings."

The French-born American microbiologist René Dubos relates what it meant to have grown up in a small French village near farms with numerous domestic animals, small woodlands, muddy ponds crowded with frogs, fields of alfalfa, wheat and sugar beets. He wrote that it was a world he could directly see, hear, smell and touch, one that provided an "enchantment that has conditioned my whole life."

After I came to know Sanchez and his family, and had lived awhile in their simple hut, he often asked me about my country. And I described it, as best I could to a man who had only been as far as Loja. Then one day Sanchez quite suddenly, without any previous explanation, surprised me by remarking, "I would like to go to your country with you."

I had not mentioned his coming to my country, but America was to him, as it was to the smallest child in the street, the greatest of dreams, the Shangri-la of their imaginations. "I would go, if we could go, as we are now—together."

I visualized Sanchez and me boarding a big plane, and flying away from the Sacred Valley, on and on, until we arrived over Manhattan and I would say, Look down below to the great city, and the Old Man would stare below and see nothing, not because he does not have eyes to see, but because New York would be enveloped in heavy dark clouds of dirt, fumes and pollution. It seemed to me that the Spanish philosopher Unamuno might have spoken the words that Sanchez, over New York, would have thought:

"Yes, yes, I see it all!" wrote Unamuno. "An enormous social activity, a mighty civilization, a profuseness of science, of art, of industry, of morality, and afterwards, when we have filled the world with industrial marvels, with great factories, with roads, museums, and libraries, we shall fall exhausted at the foot of it all, and it will subsist—for whom? Was man made for science or was science made for man?"

Sanchez, I felt, would have asked the same question. And I also felt that he would believe that his struggle atop el Chaupi, as difficult as it might be, was better than science and the city.

Some authorities on longevity have speculated that the *viejos* of Vilcabamba have added five to ten years to their lives simply by having clean air to breathe. Many medical experts, including Dr. Salvador of Quito, have observed that the quality of air in Vilcabamba promotes a longer life.

The *viejos* themselves are the first to tell you that their air is special. They could not compare their air with the heavily polluted skies of Los Angeles or Chicago, Mexico City or Tokyo. But they believe that even in Ecuador, their atmosphere is somehow special, somehow different. As one example, the Vilcabamba mayor, Celso Flavio Benitz Suarez, and I hiked to the nearby village of Malacatos, and once there, standing before a Catholic church that seemed imposing only in comparison with the squalid grouping of mud-and-stick huts around it, he turned to me:

"You see, it's a different climate here, it's more humid."

I had to agree. The air seemed heavy, and clung to one's skin as it does on an August day in Washington, D.C. One did not feel as light as in Vilcabamba where you can bounce along with a zest that makes you feel you could keep on living—"forever."

There may well be a definite connection between the air that Americans breathe and the U.S. death rate. In the United States life expectancy was constantly increasing between the early part of this century until 1960, but now, with the increase of our environmental pollution, life expectancy has begun to decrease. We carelessly have introduced chemicals into our environment without knowing the long-term effect. We are learning the results of these pesticides and pollutants the hard way. It is estimated that 85 percent of our cancer cases are caused by environmental factors. Arteriosclerosis and senility, two examples of disorders once considered irreversible and progressed in the aged, now are more widely attributed to environmental factors.

Medical experts tell us there is not a person in this country whose health would not be improved by breathing really clean air. In New York, one of the worst cities for air pollution, a doctor, Albert A. La Verne, decided to make tests on the use of pure air for therapeutic purposes. He tested 50 males and 50 females ranging in age from six to 60.

In his tests, Dr. LaVerne did a controlled experiment in which half of his hundred volunteers breathed pure air released from storage tanks during their sleeping hours, while the other half breathed the ordinary, polluted air of New York City, also compressed into tanks and released into their rooms so that none of the subjects knew which type of air he was getting. After only one night of breathing pure air most of the patients reported that they felt better. After this and a series of other studies, Dr. LaVerne concluded that polluted air "diminishes efficiency in most areas of cerebral brain functioning." In other words, if we breathe bad air we are less capable of solving our problems. The doctor also stated that the healing process itself, whether recovering from surgery or overcoming an infection, is slowed down when patients breathe badly polluted air.

In our modern urban lifestyle, many of us spend much of our time indoors, with our sprays and stale air and cooking smells.

The *viejos* on the other hand are out-of-doors most

of their lives. They get under their roofs only when they are ready for sleeping.

The *viejos* have learned to live with the rain as naturally as they do the sunshine. Once I sat talking with Señora Toledo. We were under a roof overhang of her simple mud hut. Pigs, chickens, ducks waddled in the mud, in an open courtyard. Señora Toledo wanted to feed her ducks. They were all within reach, and she could have stood under the roof and merely tossed grains out to the ducks, but she seemed deliberately intent on becoming as wet as they were.

She walked barefooted in the mud and stood in the rain, slowly dribbling out pellets of grains to the ducks. Even after she had finished her task, she stood in the rain, as apparently impervious to any deleterious effects as her ducks.

I asked, Wasn't she afraid of catching a cold in the rain?

She acted like she had never heard of the idea.

If she should get a cold, she could get over it in a few days but there is no recovery from emphysema, a respiratory disease brought on by breathing irritating substances. Physiologically, it is a loss of elasticity in the walls of the air cells of the lungs, making it difficult and sometimes impossible to expel carbon dioxide and consequently reducing the ability of the lungs to take in fresh oxygen. Symptomatically, emphysema is shortness of breath, sudden spells of coughing, mucus bubbling in the windpipe and inability to catch one's breath. Emphysema causes at least 30,000 deaths a year and is a contributory cause of another 60,000.

Dr. Arthur Levin, writing in *New York* magazine on "City Diseases that Can Kill You," listed carbon monoxide, a colorless, odorless, tasteless gas that comes from the exhaust pipes of cars, buses and other vehicles, as "probably the most dangerous surface air hazard for New Yorkers." He pointed out that "the signs of moderate monoxide poisoning can be subtle—headaches, impaired ability to think, delayed reaction time, irritability. Schoolchildren in high monoxide areas are said to have lower reading scores. The legendary irascibility of New York cabbies has been ascribed to the gas, as have the large number of taxi accidents."

Irving Selikoff, head of Mt. Sinai's environmental health unit, who produced evidence linking cancer of the lungs and abdomen with asbestos, is reported in the same magazine as saying that, "Asbestos can be filtered from New York air. Large amounts of asbestos have been found near construction sites, such as the World Trade Center, even though open-air spray-fireproofing with asbestos is now illegal in New York. Vehicle brake linings also contain asbestos, and high levels are found in the air at the entrance to the Midtown Tunnel, a site of frequent braking."

Every day we are learning more about the dust in our lungs and while the symptoms of our maladies caused by pollution may vary, everyone eventually suffers.

—In California, an association has been found between the use of pesticides and an increased death rate, the first hard evidence that pesticides affect human health.

—Studies of lung cancer deaths among white American males in 46 states showed that men who lived in urban areas had nearly two times the rate of lung cancer compared to those who lived in rural areas.

As far as is known, the air in Vilcabamba is indeed "special"—and there have been no recorded cases there of lung cancer.

5

Economics

In our capitalistic society we tend to think of money
as one of life's necessities, right along with food, clothing and shelter. It is difficult for us to imagine how we
would get food, clothing and shelter unless we had
money to pay for them.

But in addition to coins and bills there are other
means of exchange.

The Navajo Indians, for instance, with whom I
lived in 1972 on their vast reservation in the South-
west United States, initially never used money, and
even today they frequently use a barter system. One
Indian may trade sheep for a horse, or a Navajo might
exchange a handwoven rug for commodities at a trad-
ing post.

The *viejos*, like tens of thousands of "innocent,"
guileless, "primitive" people, live their lives without
money to lift them off their dirt floors, to brighten
their homes—or, one might add, to corrupt them with
the acquisitive itch.

It is difficult, if not impossible, for one who has not
lived in one of their huts, fashioned of mud and sticks,
to imagine how poor they are, by modern monetary
standards.

They are, in many cases, quite penniless.

All his life, Gabriel Sanchez has worked for a rich

hacienda owner, called a *patron.* Each day Sanchez rises at 5 A.M., and trudges to the top of the mountain to work with a hoe, or *lampa,* on a plot of corn, or *maiz.*

Under the *hacienda* system, Sanchez must work a large field for his *patron* and then he is permitted to work a small plot for himself and his family. *Peones* such as Señor Sanchez have never really known a money system, since the "master" pays in seeds, animals and the use of his land, but never with a salary.

Surviving under such a system would tax the physical strength and toughness of a man a quarter his age. But Sanchez seemed to take it in stride.

All of his water had to be brought from the San Pedro river. It was an hour's arduous trek for me, climbing from the river up the steep mountain to Sanchez' hut. At times, it was so steep that I found myself *crawling* to negotiate the incline.

On one occasion, I was at the hut and Sanchez returned from his labors to be greeted by a distraught wife, Maria Petrona, who told him the harness for the burro (the animal was old and blind) had been stolen. Without the harness the granddaughter Marie could not lead the burro up and down the steep, twisting mountain path to bring water from the river. Their lives depended on the burro and the harness.

Sanchez immediately started work on a possible solution. He gathered bits of discarded leather, only two or three inches in length, that he had saved for such an emergency, and began a tedious process of nailing these pieces together. He would somehow fashion a harness out of the "nothingness" he had at hand. I tried to talk with him, but his concentration was so intense that he blocked me out entirely. I had never seen such intensity, such concentration applied to a job. I knew his hearing was as good as mine, but now he could no longer "hear" me. All of his brain cells seemed to be applied to his one art—that of survival. His long years testified that he was good at that. Necessity demanded that he *use* his brain—or perish.

Finally, after watching him for a couple of hours at

his slow task, and knowing that it would be days or weeks before he could ever make a harness from such scraps, I asked, "Señor Sanchez, how much does a harness cost?"

"Oh, Little One, fifteen *sucres*," and he made it sound like fifteen thousand dollars.

I quickly calculated that the sum he needed was about sixty cents in our money.

I handed him some paper bills that amounted to fifteen *sucres*. They meant nothing to me (perhaps a tip for a small meal in Quito), but he thanked me as though I had paid off the mortgage of his home. Then he lit candles and prayed to *El Señor*, his God, for this miracle that had saved all of their lives. Getting up from his knees, he then prepared to walk a distance of some ten miles into the village to buy the harness.

A farm hand such as Sanchez, who is virtually "owned" by his *patron*, is neither a producer nor a consumer in the accepted sense of the words. He has nothing to sell and he can buy almost nothing.

He has coins in his pockets, in most instances, only when someone doles them out to him, perhaps a relative, a priest or a *patron*.

Sanchez must continue to work for a *patron*, because he has no other option.

Sanchez related to me that he became ill seven years ago and the *patron* said he could no longer permit Sanchez to keep a good plot of ground for himself, that he must return the plot and its harvest.

Sanchez had tears in his voice when he repeated the *patron's* words: "Get off the good land. You don't need it. You're going to die anyway—*tu vas a morir*."

I wanted to check out the story and took the bus to Loja, the provincial capital, where I visited with the *patron*, who invited me to dine with him in the Casa Blanca restaurant. He ordered French wine and filet mignons, a welcome fare in contrast to the *peon* fare I had been eating. I told the *patron* that I had been living with the *campesinos*. He laughed: "What can you learn from such poor people? They only eat roots, yucca. You'll get sick."

Then I related the story, as Sanchez had told it to me. The *patron* grew defensive: "Sanchez was no longer able to produce. I have to look after my own interests." And with bitterness and hatred in his voice the *patron* said of his 113-year-old laborer: "He is lazy." The *patron* was simply echoing an age-old credo of successful exploitation that production and earnings, not people, come first.

I went back to Vilcabamba, knowing that Sanchez could never "retire," even if he had wanted to do so. He had been allotted the most inferior, rocky plot of ground on the *hacienda* to work for himself. Work for him had become more difficult, not less so.

I thought surely that Sanchez must hate this man, and one day I asked him about this.

"No," he said, he hated the injustice done him, but not the man who meted it.

The *viejos* were like that, turning away hatred, lest they become victimized by it.

The *patron* had wronged him, but Sanchez did not feel that he had the right to take revenge. Indeed, how could he? He merely did his best, trudging daily up el Chaupi to till and coax and coddle his small plot.

"I do what I can, *hago lo que puedo*," he told me. Every day was a new struggle. As head man of his family, he still set examples of courage and work accomplishments for the others to emulate.

In many countries—in Europe, Asia, South America—I have visited in homes of the most rich and the most poor. Under every social and economic condition, I have seen that many are miserable—yet a few, like the exploited Sanchez, are never quite defeated.

The *hacienda* system interested me from the standpoint of the *viejos* and their longevity. I desired to pursue the subject to learn whether the economics of the *campesino* life had any direct bearing on the physical and psychological well-being of the Old People. In other words, had they lived long lives because of this "paternalistic" regime—or in spite of it. Dr. Alberto Avila of Quito described the *hacienda* system as "a regime that is partially paternal," and said he was inclined to believe that the "security" this regime provided was a contributing factor in the longevity of the *viejos*. The *campesinos* had no real worries, Dr. Avila maintained, since their needs would be provided. "There is a friendship between the *patron* and the working man."

When Dr. Avila spoke of a "friendship" between the *patron* and the laborer, I reminded him that the very word implies an equality, which is absent in any master-slave or *patron-peon* relationship.

Still defending the system, Dr. Avila pointed out that, "The *campesino* knows his rights and in general the *patron* respects his rights." Justice, then, would depend on the good nature, the benevolence or the whims of the wealthy landlords.

My mind couldn't put down other images, especially that of the "good" white plantation owner in the South, who bestowed a paternal kindness upon his "darkies" as he harvested the benefits of their labor. I thought of other pious overlords who applauded themselves for compassion toward their workers and of the white Americans who would give the blacks the "shirt off their backs" but not the dignity of first class citizenship status.

Contrary to Dr. Avila's contention that the *viejos* had lived a long life because of the *hacienda* system, I thought they had lived long lives in spite of it. The *viejos* were living proof that misfortunes and trials can give a meaning to life as rewarding as conditions more benign. Struggle had made them the way they were: not greedy and unburdened by the cares of money they did not possess. They were, in fact, like many "strong" black people since the period of slavery in the United States. All that they had been forced to endure made them *special*. It was a stiff price to pay, but the *viejos* like the blacks had somehow survived, their sense of morality and human decency intact.

They knew nothing of "retirement plans," annuities, or pensions. For they expected to work until the day they died. Luckily, none of the *viejos* ever, as far as I or the doctors could learn, broke a leg, so they all kept on working.

Many *viejos* have held onto the dream that the government will fulfill its promises of a better redistribution of the land, so that the soil will not be owned by only a few wealthy landlords. The agrarian reform has made a few changes in the valley. Alberto Roa, for instance, has at last obtained possession of a small plot of ground that he and his wife Sara can work for themselves, without having a master to serve. And Manuel Ramon has through the agrarian reform secured a plot of land he can call his own.

I could see the evils of the *hacienda* system and would, under no circumstances, exchange my life for the role of a *peon.* Yet, I also noted that the *viejos* had used their harsh circumstances to build strong, good characters.

They are, by their circumstances, freed from the stressful urge to accumulate money. Growth to them is a function of nature, not of stocks, portfolios or markets.

They live without the anxieties of a fluctuating Standard & Poor's index or the vagaries of the Dow Jones industrials. They are light years removed from bulls and bears, certificates of deposits and treasury bills.

They are unworried by the wild dictates of fiscal and monetary managers.

It seemed ironic that the *viejos,* among the poorest people of the world, would worry less about money and possessions than the richest people in the world. The English writer C. P. Snow observed, "I have never in my life seen Europeans so concerned about money as they are today." Those who have money hope to get more, to buy more "security." The *viejos* never think of money that way.

Once I asked the gentle, generous Señor Ramon, "What would he like most to have in this world?"

He thought a long while without answering, and then I asked specifically, "Would he like to have money?"

"No," he said, simply, "I have no need for it."

He is the same *viejo* who had described the meaning of his life as death. Money obviously would not help in that land beyond the grave.

6

Eating the Vilcabamba Way

The idea of a planned diet would seem ridiculous to
the *viejos* of Vilcabamba. They literally live from
meal to meal. If you ask one how long he wants to
live, he replies, with the fatalism common to the very
old, "One more day."

Necessity gives everything they eat a certain
primitive freshness. They do not horde food for a tomorrow that may never come. They have neither the
means nor the resources to stock a larder. They
have nothing remotely comparable to a food store or
market, as we know them, with selections of packaged and canned goods. I never saw any canned foods
in any of the homes, nor did I ever see a housewife
open a package of breakfast cereal, pancake mix, or
crackers. Processed food is virtually unknown to the
viejos.

They cook only a small amount, enough to satisfy
appetites accustomed to scarcity. Rarely if ever are
there leftovers. Even in what might pass for a restaurant or a boardinghouse, the *señoras* will serve
meals only if they have bought the ingredients that
same day. They cook one pot of boiled corn, called
mote, or one pot of rice, and when that is gone they
will not prepare more. Unless you go early you will
find all the food has been eaten. Without refrigera-

tion, they can store very little that is perishable. Milk is a precious commodity, and only a small quantity, fresh from the cow, is sold each morning. The eggs available, which are scarce also, are freshly laid. Vegetables are picked fresh from the gardens, their nutritional value intact. Fruits are plucked the same day and often eaten on the spot. Such a diet is blessedly free of the artificial preservatives or additives injected into so many foods in the United States, which increasingly concern health authorities and dietitians.

Processing, among other natural occurrences, can reduce and destroy the nutrient content in food. Robert S. Harris, Ph.D., of the Department of Nutrition and Food Science at the Massachusetts Institute of Technology, wrote that by the time processed foods reach you, "they may have been shipped and stored, trimmed, blanched, frozen, canned, condensed, dehydrated, pasteurized, sterilized, smoked, cured, milled, roasted, cooked, toasted or puffed. What's left of their composition after any combination of those tortures is then liable to be further stolen by heat, light, oxygen, oxalates, antivitamins, acidity, alkalinity, metal catalysts, enzymes and irradiation."

But the abuse of natural foods may have only begun. "Some chemical and pharmaceutical companies are making large investments in artificial hams, artificial cheeses, and similar new types of foods," according to Dr. Alexander M. Schmidt of the Food and Drug Administration. By 1980, he said, two-thirds of all the food we Americans eat will have been previously prepared outside the home. In the mid-seventies the figure was about 50 percent.

The *viejos* of Vilcabamba have always eaten the most natural of diets: wild game, wild berries, nuts, whole grains, vegetables, fruits. In his book, *Nutrition and Physical Degeneration*, Dr. Weston Price said he had found pockets of healthy, long-living people among diverse races of people in every corner of the world, in the tropics, the Arctic region, some in mountains, some on small islands. They had two things in common: they ate natural diets and enjoyed superb health. He concluded that it did not matter whether people ate primarily a grain diet, a meat and fish diet, a dairy diet or a combination of the three, so long as what they ate was *fresh* and *whole*.

The people of Vilcabamba, isolated behind their comfortable mountains, were not familiar with our national preoccupation with obesity and our attendant obsession with calories, carbohydrates, protein and fats. They found it difficult to believe that the richest people in the world would come to study the diet of some of the poorest people in the world, as if their simple fare consisted of secrets beyond the reach of wealth and influence.

By our standards of abundance the people ate a "poor" diet in variety, as well as quantity. In any one day, for example, you could go to a corner supermarket and see on view a greater variety of foods, from soup to sweets, in greater quantity than would be available in Vilcabamba for years. However, because the *viejos* eat the entire food—the bran of their grain, the skin of their fruit and vegetables (and they suffer no danger of sprays or chemicals)—they are able to get real nutrition from a relatively simple diet. We in the United States cannot depend on this, even if we eat "right" because so much food value is lost in our modern methods of cultivation, processing, packaging and storage.

It would be difficult for a simple farm worker or *campesino* to comprehend that, in the United States, a man may be twenty pounds overweight and still be badly nourished, which indeed is often the case.

The *viejos* were constantly puzzled by questions about their diet. Each time I asked a villager what he or she liked to eat for breakfast, lunch or dinner, the response was the same: "Whatever is at hand—*Lo que hay.*"

Here was a clear case of "poor" people eating the cheapest, simplest foods and absorbing more nutrition than many affluent folks. My friend Roscoe

Dixon had told a story about black slaves in the southern United States being given all "leftovers," such as "pot likker" drained from collards and throw-away beef bones, gizzards, hearts and liver. "And the slaves were getting stronger and the plantation owner was getting weaker." The rich often have thrown out the nutritious elements when they discarded organ meats, bones and the water in which vegetables were cooked.

Once I asked Micaela Quezada, whose reputed age was 104, "What is your diet?"

"Poor man's food, *la comida de los pobres*," she replied.

Señorita Quezada invited me to stay for supper one evening. I sat on a small stool while she busied herself building a fire. She somehow projected height, and her movements were surprisingly agile. She loved to punctuate her talk with theatrical gestures, and I could visualize her, under different circumstances, as an actress. She was indeed enacting a role, that of a woman in her kitchen. It occurred to me that growing old for this woman, despite her poverty, was easier than those aging in the idle comfort of nursing homes and sanitoria, their minds turned inward to loneliness and creeping despair with their every "need" supplied by others. This plain, simple woman remained forever busy with her hands, with the myriad tasks of taking care of herself, building fires, preparing food, making do.

As I looked around, I was impressed by the spartan environment. This was not a kitchen, as we know it; it was only a corner of the room, with an iron stove and a few sparse sticks of firewood. The average housewife, who keeps a reserve of food in her pantry, could not imagine the nothingness of the Vilcabamba cupboard. Actually, there are no cupboards in the huts. Señorita Quezada had one shelf near her iron stove, and it contained only a small can for cooking fat. Nothing else. No sugar. No salt or pepper shakers, no mustard, spices, ketchup, Worcestershire sauce or ready mixes. In short, none of the condiments we deem indispensable in preparing our meals.

The señorita's room opened to a small patio or courtyard. I could see a pig roaming freely, a few ducks and in one corner the little guinea pigs or *cuis* that look like giant rats. Señorita Quezada wanted to honor me by offering me the finest. "You like *cuis?*" I looked at the rodent-like animals. I imagined my eating "rat"—as that was what I always "saw" when I saw a *cui*. Still, having been raised on a Texas Panhandle diet of clabber, tripe, black-eyed peas and buttermilk, I thought that I could digest whatever the señorita served me. I also knew, however, that to her palate, a *cui* was a succulent delicacy, like a hundred-year-old egg to a Chinese epicure. I told her that I would be delighted with something *simple*. I knew that would be maize, potatoes or a bowl of soup, which suited me fine. She had a pot boiling, and I learned it was her favorite dish, a soup made from beef bones, *caldo de hueso*. I asked her, just how had she made it, what were the ingredients she had used?

She hesitated to give her recipe. Why wouldn't she tell me? I asked. She said it was the same as my asking her to tell how she put her clothes on each morning; she had always done it, but had never had to stop and tell anyone *how*.

The centenarians are known to have healthy bones. I did not see anyone disabled or limping. Nor did I ever hear of any of the Old People falling and breaking an arm, leg or hip. The nutrients from bones that Señorita Quezada got in her soup are rich in calcium which is linked to a healthy heart and circulatory system, and it also strengthens one's bones against the fractures of an aging body.

Today in the cities many people add a bone meal supplement to their diets. Bone meal contains calcium, phosphorus and potassium as well as copper, iron, manganese, zinc, boron, flourine, iodine and sulphur.

Almost all foods contain at least some calcium, inasmuch as it is a vital component in the physiology of plants and animals. However, when we refine grains, such as wheat and rice, we reduce the calcium content. Instant rice, for example, has about one-fifth the calcium value of whole brown rice. When it comes to meat, about 99 percent of the animal's calcium is stored in the bones and teeth. The rich man who eats a filet mignon is missing some of the nutrients that Señorita Quezada gets in her bone soup, "a poor man's diet."

The first time I heard Micaela Quezada use the phrase, "a poor man's diet," I thought it sounded like a title for a good cookbook. And possibly it would sell in the United States. Fat people are "hungry" to hear all that they can eat to get slim. We are all activists, and will *eat* almost any given diet, but what we will not do is what they do in Vilcabamba —eat very little.

Lunch is the most important meal. Generally the *campesino* doesn't come home for lunch. He eats in the place where he is working. He might take his lunch with him, or someone takes it to him, or at the *hacienda* where he is working he might be given food.

Even though lunch is the most important meal, it is relatively frugal.

We in the United States get a caloric surplus even from a seemingly reasonable diet. Our excess poundage comes from our modern living: inactivity, a superabundance of attractive, high-calorie foods and an emphasis on consumption. For calorie-conscious Americans, it will not seem surprising that nutrition experts attribute a great deal to the fact that the *viejos* are not gourmands. Dr. Guillermo Vela of the University of Quito and one of his country's leading experts on nutrition believes that "the longevity and health of the centenarians is due as much to what they do not eat as to what they eat."

Dr. Vela said that obesity actually is an energy

crisis in reverse. Its fundamental cause is the consumption of more calories than the body uses up. Whether the excess calories are in the form of protein, fat or carbohydrate, they are all converted to fat and stored in the body's fat depots.

Of the old people in Vilcabamba, Dr. Vela said, "You will see that the people are very well developed, they are thin, but this is not a malady, obesity is an illness. They are thin, but they give the impression of very good health, good nutrition."

Overweight persons have an increased risk of developing diabetes, heart disease, high blood pressure and chronic respiratory disorders, all of which tend to shorten their lives. They also suffer to an abnormal degree from such problems as back and foot aches. "Contrary to what many think," Dr. Vela said, "exercise does not make a person so hungry that he eats even more than he normally would. In fact, exercise has a 'euphoriant effect' that diminishes the tendency to turn to food for emotional satisfaction."

I myself experienced this in Vilcabamba. Walking up and down mountains, the *viejos* and I never stopped to talk about food. Our minds were occupied with love stories or other thoughts more interesting than food. And when we sat down to eat, everyone was courteous, and still more interested in talking than eating. I never saw anyone greedy for food. Or afraid he would not get his share. I never saw any *viejo* overeat. I saw families with one plate of maize to share who were less greedy than a group of *gringos* eating a five-course meal. I ate less because they were a good influence.

Dr. Vela said the average daily diet in Vilcabamba provides 1,200 calories. Then he added that Americans of all ages have an average daily intake of 3,300 calories.

The breakdown graphically illustrated the disparity between the average intake in Vilcabamba and the United States:

CALORIES	Vilcabamba	1,200
	United States	3,300
PROTEINS	Vilcabamba	35 to 38
	United States	100
FAT	Vilcabamba	16
	United States	157
CARBOHYDRATES	Vilcabamba	200–250
	United States	380

Dr. Vela pointed out that "people in the United States eat almost three times as many calories, three times as many proteins, and almost ten times as much fat.

"We have to make a campaign to show this. This is what is killing people, attacking their hearts. The food consumption figures are *quotas extraordinarias*. We must teach more moderation."

I saw no more than two or three overweight people in the Sacred Valley—and they were not *viejos*. In the States, by contrast, every other person I see needs to shed excess fat. My Washington friend Mollye commented, "When I see people crossing the street, or when I see tourists walking out of the White House, I think: Why are so many so fat!" Statistics bear out our impressions: fifty percent of our population is said to be overweight.

The centenarians of Vilcabamba reminded me of the Greek Stoic Epictetus who in A.D. 94 said a man should behave in life as he would at a banquet, taking only a polite portion of what is offered. We Americans go to cocktail parties and banquets and nibble at and consume abundant portions of everything in sight. The midnight snack is not an uncommon cap to an evening of gorging. I myself think of food almost constantly in the United States, and I am fairly typical. This is all the more curious, with the activities and diversions here. In Vilcabamba I had nothing to do but hike up mountains and talk with Old People, and yet my mind never dwelled on food. I wasn't frustrated, I didn't yearn for chocolate. It may be that their unavailability had disciplined my appetite. One doesn't reach into a void for a candy bar. But I suspected other reasons for this absence of the usual cravings. The stress was missing. The struggle was reduced to elementary requirements. Traffic never jangled my nerves, and decisions about food were simply unnecessary. No compulsions were generated by the bombardment of television commercials exhorting me to bite into a particular brand of potato chips. In the Sacred Valley the appetite was reduced to a monastic dimension.

Many people in the United States live alone, whereas I never met anyone who lived alone in Vilcabamba. In this country, those who live alone often eat alone, undiverted by conversation or companionship. They compensate by overeating. I remembered a talk with a retired Baltimore resident now living in Florida who told me he was 60 and a widower for several years, and that he no longer had sex. He was afraid to approach a woman, afraid she would rebuff him. So, I asked, What was the most important thing in his life?

"Eating," he said.

I repeated the story to Dr. Vela, who said, "For many people a meal represents the highest pleasure. Many are alone, without family, all they have is to eat. The fat person has a psychological problem."

We have "everything" here at home, including psychological problems that are unknown in Vilcabamba.

Once I invited Señorita Quezada to my second-floor sleeping quarters over the Churo store, and she was as excited as my mother when I took her to the top of the Empire State Building. The trip up the one flight of stairs to my loft was as high as Micaela had ever been. We sat on my small cot and talked. Since she was impressed by her trip to the second-story loft, I told her about men going to the moon.

"You don't say! *Que tal!*" she responded.

But she was not impressed. Up was up, and high, high up was not that special. Her feet were quite earthbound. Like any woman, she enjoyed seeing the living arrangement of another woman. So, now she knew where I slept. And then she was more curious about how I lived back home. What, for instance, she asked, did I eat? Did I eat maize and *frijoles* back home?

I nodded in agreement.

"Well," she added, "was that all? Was there any other food, *algun mas?*"

Yes, I told her. And pictures of huge supermarkets, and well-stocked pantries and overcrowded restaurants, sometimes four to a city block, came to my mind. I would never be able to explain our abundance to this simple woman. But, I wanted to try.

I then told her many people suffered a desire to eat too much food. I said we had so many fat people they joined clubs such as "Weight Watchers" to report to each other what they had eaten, and that they helped each other eat less.

She listened incredulously. Old people in Vilcabamba could not imagine spending hours talking about the yucca, the yams, the corn that they ate. To her, our overwhelming interest in food was more astonishing than men landing on the moon.

No one really knows what causes obesity.

"Obesity is a symptom, not a disease," said Dr. Myron Winick, director of the Columbia University's Institute of Human Nutrition. Dr. Jean Mayer, Harvard University nutritionist and longtime student of the causes of obesity, said, "Attributing overweight to overeating is hardly more illuminating than ascribing alcoholism to alcohol." The obvious solution, according to Dr. Mayer, is to move more. "Walk, don't ride. Take the stairs, not the elevator," he recommends. Doctors say most of the ten billion dollars worth of ill-conceived reducing schemes that the obese in our country buy each year only further compromise their health.

To break down and analyze the diet of the cen-

tenarians is to encounter some contradictions and
myths of modern nutrition. For example, we generally consider meat and fish as indispensable sources
of protein. The *viejos*, however, *eat very little meat*.
They get the bulk of their protein from vegetables,
even though they are far from being vegetarians.
Beans, a staple of their diet, provide a rich source
of protein. Also, they eat many cereals such as corn,
wheat, barley; and vegetables such as lettuce, car-
rots, turnips; and tubers, such as potatoes, yucca and
sweet potatoes, or *camotes*.

Dr. Vela said many affluent people forgot that
beans were a good source of proteins. "You can get
proteins from beans as well as from meat," he emphasized.

We also get proteins from dairy products and
Dr. Vela thought the Americans' habit of drinking
enriched milk, pouring heavy cream on cereals and
eating ice cream also enriched our history of heart
and artery problems. He said we should think of
milk as a "food" not a beverage. "Consider how the
people in the United States drink milk. Everyone!
And it's milk of the first quality. As for us, we have
products of less quality or cream content, whereas
in the United States it is all of the first quality. You
don't need this extra fat and cholesterol. This is what
is killing the people.

"I've given up milk entirely. Adults don't need
milk," he told me.

Better, he suggested, yogurt, cottage cheese, and
a simple bland white cheese that I ate often in Vilcabamba. It seemed to be the Old Peoples' equivalent
of yogurt that is consumed among many long-living
people in other parts of the world, such as Turkey,
Arabia, Russia and Hunza.

While the Vilcabamba *viejos* have always gotten
most of their proteins from beans and vegetables,
with very little meat added to their dishes, we in
the United States have expected beef to satisfy our
protein requirements. Dr. Vela, as have many dietary
authorities, said that the concentration of animal fats

adds cholesterol and can contribute to many heart and vascular diseases in the United States.

Being penny poor, the *viejos* eat the cheapest cuts of meat, pig's tails, also lung, heart, brains, tongue, liver, sweetbreads, tripe, gizzards and liver. I had eaten many of these cheap cuts as a child. Growing up during the depression days, I often was sent to the grocery store, a nickel clutched in one hand, and I would tell the grocer, "Give me five cents' worth of liver." And I would take home enough meat for six people. In those days, the butcher gave soup bones away and sold two pounds of liver for five cents. We in this country consume vast quantities of dessicated beef liver and beef bone meal tablets, both of which the people of Vilcabamba get the natural way.

In my childhood we ate meat on a special day, such as Sunday, but never every day of the week. Now many people in this country eat bacon for breakfast, a hamburger for lunch and steak for dinner. Beef has become such a prestige food of our affluent society that consumption has jumped from 1952's 62 pounds per person to 116 pounds per person in the 1970s.

The two heart specialists, Dr. Salvador and Dr. Avila, as well as Dr. Vela, all thought that the low quantity of animal fats in the Vilcabamba diet was a possible clue to the dietary strength of the *viejos*. Dr. Avila, for instance, said, "When you go to the supermarket a lot of what you buy is filled with fats. You might eat pork two or three times in the week, as, for example, bacon for breakfast. But in their case they raise pigs strictly as a business. One family may have one pig, raise it and sell it. They might have pork once, as a celebration, but it is nothing they would eat every day.

"And they never eat butter. They can't afford it. It is just not available."

I knew from firsthand experience he was right. I had never seen butter, or any substitute, in a *casa* during my entire stay in Vilcabamba. Their lack of refrigeration would make it difficult to keep, even if they could afford it. Dr. Vela had stressed, "In Ecuador, we eat very little fat. I speak of the big majority. Within a small group of *ricos* they might eat a lot of fat and butter, but these will be the ones who must go to a doctor. My figures are for the general population."

In the pockets of longevity in Hunza in West Pakistan, and Russia, the long-living people get many of their carbohydrates from an enriched, homemade bread, but Vilcabamba people eat little bread. "*Poco pan*," Dr. Vela noted. "The centenarians get unrefined carbohydrates found in beans, and whole grain corn, wheat, barley, and vegetables and tubers, potatoes, yucca, yams."

I had always thought that eating carbohydrates were what piled on the weight. I knew that while in Vilcabamba I ate a lot of boiled corn called *mote* and beans, I felt fine and I lost weight. Dr. Vela said these two items were the main source of the Vilcabamba carbohydrates. Dr. Vela said, "The *longevos* were lucky in that for most of their lives they avoided white sugar. It not only has been stripped of its value but it actually drains resources from other foods in an average diet."

Dr. Vela found few fat people in the Sacred Valley. I was with him once when he interviewed a stout woman of forty-five who had given birth to 15 children, 11 of them living. "I got married at 19, and all of my children were large," she related. She admitted that she had a sweet tooth, and Dr. Vela asked if she bought white sugar. She admitted that she did.

Until recently, all the Old People ate only unrefined brown sugar called *panela*, as well as molasses, both of which are rich in zinc and iron. Now, more "civilized," they buy the white sugar not realizing that the good has been processed out of the *panela* and that the sucrose itself doesn't help anyone.

I could see the good dietary habits of the Old People changing before my eyes. Once a friend, Manuel Pardo, and I hiked up a mountain to visit his sister Sara and her husband Alberto Roa, all vigorous, alert people in their nineties.

After a simple evening meal, the *señora* served us coffee, and when I put the cup to my lips, the *señora* and Pardo and the others all shouted "No! No!" and motioned me, as if I were drinking poison, to put down the cup. The *señora* spooned white sugar into my coffee, and then I was allowed to drink it. They were "honoring" me by giving me the white sugar. The *viejos* like other people of the world are adopting our habit of liking white sugar and it will, of course, do them no good. They were better off with their crude blocks of brown *panela*.

Just as one example, older people especially are likely to have low body levels of chromium, and some doctors have linked low chromium levels to bad arteries. Refined sugar and refined flour have a great deal of their chromium removed, whereas whole grain flour is a good source of chromium, and natural forms of sugar that have not been processed also contain reasonable amounts.

Many nutritionists tell us today we would do well to eliminate refined sugar and refined flour from our diets. Dr. Weston Price, who wrote that a natural diet was the first rule for superb health, said wherever processed foods, particularly white flour and sugar, were introduced to healthy communities, the people's health soon showed signs of deterioration.

Dr. Otto Schaefer, who studied the health of Eskimos, believes sugar and other processed foods are the direct cause of an enormous increase in rotten teeth, arteriosclerosis, obesity, gallbladder disease and other pathological conditions familiar to many Americans but, until recently, rare among Eskimos.

When the most healthy of the *viejos* of Vilcabamba wanted the sweet taste, they added some fresh fruit such as bananas, *naranjillas* (a small fruit, a type of orange), papayas or mangos to their diet, or they poured honey on fresh bland, white cheese, *queso con miel*. The dessert as we know it does not exist in Vilcabamba. In all my visits to many different

homes, I never saw any kind of "sweets" or dessert.
I did not see a single cake or pie, torte, custard, gela-
tin. Ice cream, of course, was unthinkable.

After my initial visit to Vilcabamba, I went to Fort
Worth to visit my mother and my sister Margaret,
who gave a small country club dinner party to
which she invited the writer, John Howard Griffin
and his wife Piedy. Griffin once lived in France and
is a gourmet cook, and he and Piedy both enjoy rich
cream caramel custards and French chocolate mous-
ses, as who among us doesn't.

When it came time to eat our desserts, we
were choosing from a vast array of cheesecakes,
strawberry tarts and chocolate covered Napoleons,
and several of us, not being able to choose one,
took two. Mother observed, "Grace says the people in
Vilcabamba never have desserts," and Piedy, laughing, rejoined, "Who wants to live so long?"

Dr. Alex Comfort had said as much when he observed that, "If longevity requires tiresome and
lifelong diet restrictions, our foods suggest that
we don't value longevity highly enough to make
ourselves uncomfortable."

Rather, I think our choice of foods suggests, not
that we don't value health and longevity, but that,
unlike the *viejos*, we in the United States are victims
of a constant barrage of advertising that sells us on
the idea that "rich" gooey, junk desserts, constantly displayed in our supermarkets, in magazines,
newspapers and on TV, will satisfy us physically and
emotionally, when the opposite is true.

The *viejos*, Dr. Vela suggests, choose the best
"sweet"—a piece of fresh fruit. And in the Sacred Valley you can select from among the most delicious
fruits in the world. I especially liked the papayas,
mangoes, bananas, pineapple, figs, *naranjillas*, wa-
termelons and oranges. Oranges were one of the
most plentiful fruits in Vilcabamba. A *viejo* who
seemingly had "nothing" could always find an orange
to give me as a present.

The people ate many oranges, and with these

and other fresh fruit they got all the vitamin C they
needed, as well as the other nutritional richness of
fresh fruit, including energy from the fruit sugar.
Vitamin C helps prevent colds and other infections,
builds up health of the skin, and makes the "glue"
that holds the body's cells together.

Some doctors tell us that vitamin C should play a
prominent role in the "nutrition first" approach to
arthritis. Many aged persons in our country, particularly those in institutions, eat little fruit and have
correspondingly low levels of vitamin C.

The biochemist Dr. Roger J. Williams has stressed
that we are all different people and that our needs
vary individually. Each of the *viejos* had favorite
foods. Alberto Roa, 90, who was married to Manuel
Pardo's sister, Sara, looked and acted as if he were no
more than 60. Roa touted the virtues of eggs. He
said when he was young he worked hard, *muy duro*,
on a *hacienda*. He got up at 4:30 A.M. and for his
breakfast he ate eight soft-boiled eggs, beaten together in a glass.

I looked in disbelief, repeating his figure eight,—
"*¿Ocho?*"

He replied, "*Si,* and sometimes twelve, *doce.*"

Pardo's wife Sara said her favorite meal was a
bowl of cooked oats with milk. She said it was nutritious and if she ate it at night it enabled her to
sleep soundly.

Oatmeal has always been my favorite breakfast because I had eaten it as a "poor" child during the depression. I was amazed that when I had money in
my purse and found myself in Paris or New York,
studying impressive breakfast menus, and telling
myself to eat what I pleased, I discovered that what
I liked most of all was a bowl of oatmeal. Numerous
others feel this way too.

In his book *An Illustrated History of the Olym-
pics,* Richard Schaap reported that Paavo Nurmi, the
fabulous distance runner who won seven gold medals
in three Olympic Games, reportedly ate black bread

and fish, but one day a reporter followed the Flying
Finn and learned that Nurmi's favorite dish was really oatmeal.

Once, I invited Manuel Pardo, 96, to the el Violente,
just about the only *casa* that bears the name of a
restaurant, and we ordered lunch, *comida*. On this
day it was the root, yucca, with some pig meat.
The meat was so tough he took his own large butcher knife from a side holster to cut it.

"Do you eat much pig?" I asked.

"I eat anything."

He didn't eat much yucca. "It fattens you." He
gave some of the yucca to a dog lying at his feet.

"Are you afraid of fat?" I asked.

"I have fear of nothing, *de nada*." Again and again,
the old people said, "I eat *anything*."

I noted that Dr. Vela ate precisely the way he
preached: very wisely. Forty-five, enthusiastic, energetic, humorous, he admitted that formerly he was
fat,—"I was called *el gordo Vela*." He slimmed
down, eating the Vilcabamba way.

I asked Vela what he ate for breakfast.

"A cup of coffee, no cream or sugar. And fresh
cheese, nothing else, *nada mas*."

He had already told me he never drank milk.
"And butter?"

"Never."

"And cream?"

"*Nunca*."

"And your lunch?"

"This is a very good meal. I start with a soup, a
potato soup or a vegetable soup. A piece of meat, a
little rice. And dessert of fruit. A drink, usually before lunch. It could be a whiskey, a gin or a du-
bonnet—whatever, *cualquier cosa*."

"And bread?"

"*Si, un pan*. And at night, almost the same kind of
meal, but less than at noon."

"And sometimes beer or wine? Some drinking?"

"*Si*. Generally at end of week. I have a large

family, a brother who is an archbishop of the church, we have big family reunions at the end of the week, and we take drinks."

"What is your general advice about nutrition and health?"

"Get a weight that is normal, and even below normal. Be careful about animal fats . . . and proteins, also.

"Eat *little meat. Less* of proteins, less fat . . . nothing in excess of nature.

"And, *less* carbohydrates."

I asked what he had learned from Vilcabamba.

"*I am convinced that the less the people eat the better off they are.* Without going to extremes, it seems to me that a diet that is balanced—without excesses of any kind—is one of the secrets of health in this life.

"Consider that the insurance companies know that obesity and high blood pressure are the two things that worry them most of all.

"Diet is a very important aspect. And because we eat, all of the days, we are following the right rules, or breaking them."

In Quito, I ate several times in the home of Dr. Salvador and his wife Consuelo. They are both gourmet cooks and served marvelous dinners, the type you can find in Paris, along with superb wines. Dr. Salvador and I have the same philosophy. He phrased it this way: "Don't always say no to life. Nor, always yes. Live, enjoy."

7

Smoking and Drinking

Ecuadorian medical authorities who were early visitors to the Sacred Valley offered cigarettes and liquor
to the *viejos*, and were apparently surprised to learn
that they accepted their gifts. Actually, though, most
of the *viejos* are not habitual smokers, and rarely
have anything alcoholic to drink.

Most of these early visitors did not stay overnight in the village itself, and so did not come to
know the *viejos* on an intimate, day-to-day basis and
had no concrete evidence of their real habits.

At the suggestion of a Quito doctor, who himself
likes to smoke, I took the *viejos* presents of cigarettes. Carpio, Erazo, Ramon, Sanchez and others accepted them graciously, and occasionally one lit
up a cigarette in my presence and smoked it, but
after living in their huts with them, I learned that,
with two or three exceptions, none of the *viejos*
smoked regularly.

They are perhaps the most disciplined people I
have ever known. They are, however, individualists,
so that like the rest of us, their group ranged from
those who boasted that they drank and smoked heavily in their youth to those who were completely abstemious and righteously asserted that they had
never been stained by nicotine or scarred by alcohol.

None of the women I came to know did any smoking or drinking. This was true in the case of such old women as Señoras Toledo, Sanchez, Ramon and Roa, with whom I lived in the valley. The influence of the Catholic church was dominant in their lives. They were taught that while some men might be allowed to take certain liberties, such as smoking and drinking, they as women could not without incurring the harsh disapproval of their society. It would not be good for their souls—nor the health of their children. Women were, in short, taught to be "pure" in body and spirit. In latino countries women have, for the most part, abided by these injunctions.

I became convinced that the *viejos'* longevity stemmed in a major way from their disciplined habits, the absence of harmful indulgences. As a matter of fact, the struggle to exist left most of them few alternatives.

Being poor *campesinos,* working for wealthy landlords, imposed a certain discipline in itself. This, however, did not prevent many of the old men from recalling the "wild oats" they had sown in their youth. Today, they were different. They had lived through their youth, when as Pardo once put it, "You want to try everything." Now, strong drink was not important to them. And neither were cigarettes. Many of the old men would, however, enjoy taking an occasional drink.

Once Sanchez was in the village and I asked him to have a drink with me. The *viejos* always appreciate an invitation. They know how to receive, and feel that they have no right to refuse when you make a gesture of friendship. We sat outside a *casa* where a Señora Cueca sold food and drink from her own kitchen. I suggested a homemade liquor, asking Sanchez:

"Would you like a glass of *aguardiente?*"

He said he would.

But the señora had none.

"What about beer," I asked Sanchez.

"Oh, si." He liked *cerveza*.

The señora had none.

We settled for two bottles of sweetened cherry pop.

I watched Sanchez turn the bottle to his lips and drink from it with an expression of deep satisfaction, the kind a Frenchman might have in tasting a rare, vintage wine. Some studies show that thousands of old people in our land suffer from dying taste buds. They complain that nothing they drink or eat tastes good anymore. Obviously, Sanchez did not have this affliction. He relished every swallow of the soft drink. I found it awful and almost unpalatable. When he finished his king-sized bottle, I passed mine over to him. He thanked me and again drank with genuine pleasure. I could not imagine his relishing either *aguardiente* or *cerveza* more than he had the sweetened soda water.

Life had been reduced to its basics. He was thirsty. There was drink. The kind of drink did not matter to this simple, undemanding man. For him it was a moment to relax, a respite from hard labor.

In the days that I spent with Sanchez and his family in their mountain hut I never saw any of them take a drink of liquor. They lived a frugal existence. They had no money to spend. And they kept no liquor of any kind in the hut. However, Sanchez had a son in the village who worked as custodian in the church. I had on occasion seen him "stumbling drunk." Drinking is, in fact, now a problem in the village, but the excessive drinkers are the young and middle-aged, not the *viejos*.

Miguel Carpio, whose estimated age was 110 to 127, according to the doctors who visited the valley, was always boastful of his past. He had, he would tell you with a twinkle in his eyes, really lived a full life, and he meant it as most men would. He had played hard, he had worked hard. He had known countless women and in his youth he had drunk much *aguardiente* and smoked many cigarettes. Occasionally he still smokes, perhaps one cigarette a week, no more. Once, while I was visiting him, he lit a cigarette, his hand steady as a youth's.

"I like it, *me gusta*," he said, as we sat talking. But although I had given him an entire carton, I did not see him smoking any more of the cigarettes. I later learned he gave them to a grandson.

By way of contrast, there were the wholly abstemious ones. For example, Alberto Roa, 91, condemned smoking and drinking as terrible vices, and insisted that he had lived to a healthy old age because he had been a teetotaler. He also said, with a touch of self-righteousness, that he remained a virgin until he was 30 and had never touched any woman but his wife, Sara.

On one occasion, Sara's brother, Manuel Pardo, sat listening to Roa's account of his pristine habits, and it was plain he had heard the litany many times. Finally Pardo interjected, "I've smoked and drank, and had so many women I couldn't count them. And I'm five years older than you." Pardo's boast had a tinge of disgust for Roa's professed virtues.

Once I heard Erazo and Celso Leon, who said he was 105, discuss longevity in terms of their personal habits. Leon related that he had never smoked, never drank and never chased women, "I was always faithful, *fiel*, to my wife." Erazo chuckled, and said that was no recipe for a good, rich, ripe old age. "I've lived longer than you," he told Leon—and then launched into a recital of the *aguardiente* he had drunk and all the beautiful women, *mujeres bonitas*, he had known.

I often visited with one chain-smoker, Angel Modesto Burneo V., who had a red beard and bright clear green eyes that usually seemed to be laughing at his own jokes. One day I was sitting beside him on a bench outside his stucco house. Mariada, nine, and Nancy Venitas, ten, two village children, came by to chat. As the young girls, shy and full of giggles, stood before us, Modesto turned and winked at me, and in

a soft aside for my ears only, indicating that he and
I shared many hidden secrets, observed: "Their hearts
are pure. Not like yours and mine."

Modesto has lived his ninety-one years, mistakes
and all, with a vigorous defiance of the conventional
health rules. He readily admits he was a heavy drinker and he's been a heavy smoker, thirty to forty
cigarettes a day, since he was eighteen.

Usually, when we sat on the bench, talking, Modesto had a large pan of tobacco beside him, and pieces
of toilet paper in which he busily rolled the tobacco
to make limp and scraggly cigarettes that he sold to
villagers.

"How many cigarettes," I asked Modesto, "could
he roll in a day?"

"Two thousand, more or less."

"Two thousand," I echoed in amazement.

"Others make four thousand in a day," he said.

"I take the tobacco leaves from the plant and let
them dry in honey or molasses," Modesto explained.
"It's half-dried tobacco. And when you inhale, it
takes a great effort, a grand *fuerza*, because the tobacco does not light up well."

And smoking was not bad for his health? I asked.

"No. And that's because I don't inhale. This is what
is bad, because the nicotine would stay in your
lungs." He demonstrated as he talked, repeatedly
saying he took the smoke in and blew it out his nose,
without the tobacco passing through his lungs. I
watched his demonstration carefully, but I was un-
able to judge whether smoke entered into his lungs.
Later Dr. Leaf told me that tests showed that this
could be done. He added, however, that, "It is very
unusual for someone who is a regular cigarette smoker not to inhale."

Modesto had a friend, Pasto Abarca, who made the
liquor, *aguardiente*. One day Modesto and I visited
Abarca, 76, who was slightly built, with thick jet
black hair. Abarca owned a small store where he sold
hand-rolled cigarettes and homemade *aguardiente*.

To make the *aguardiente,* which literally translates—
"fire water"—he had a crude still operation, with
sugar cane fermenting in tin wash tubs.

"I wake up each morning at 5 A.M. I can't sleep,"
he told me. "So I get up. And the first thing I do is
take a strong drink of *aguardiente.*" He agreed to
demonstrate the process for fermenting sugar cane in
tin wash tubs to produce alcohol, of the *primer paso.*
I had previously tasted an *aguardiente* that was processed in a plant. But this was a cruder, more simple
home-still operation, and could not be called "processed" liquor.

Abarca poured drinks in tin cups for Modesto and
me. I saw that it was colorless, like water. When I
sipped, I felt a tingling sensation I had felt with
strong, undiluted vodka.

Dr. Leaf, in his visit to the Caucasus Mountains in
Russia, said he found several examples of centenarians who continued to smoke and drink. He recalled
that Khafaf Lasuria, "More than 130 years old, unabashedly admitted to keeping a bottle of vodka in
her room and to taking a little nip every morning
before breakfast. She drank wine throughout my visit
with her. She also smokes and inhales at least one
package of cigarettes every day, a habit she said she
started in 1910, after her brother, who was some 10
years younger than she, died at age 60. . . . She was,
however, already 70 when she took up the habit!"

The smoking and drinking habits of Khafaf Lasuria
have been widely publicized, in photos released by
the Soviet press, but actually her age was never veri-
fied by sources that scientists elsewhere could un-
equivocally accept. And, since Dr. Leaf's visit, the
remarkable old woman has died, so that the secret of
her "true age" probably died with her.

While several long-living people of the Caucasus
Mountains smoke, almost none of the long-living people of Hunza, in the Indian subcontinent, do. As
Dr. Leaf points out, "They don't grow the tobacco
and they don't have any money to buy it."

Dr. Leaf observed that even if a few centenarians

n remote areas have smoked to excess, they were exceptional cases that would give none of us any guarantees that we, too, could smoke and live to the century mark. He said some smokers and some tobacco companies were attempting to show that it is not the tobacco as such that is causing cancers and other maladies, but a personality trait among smokers. One of the exponents of this theory, a scientist who likes to chain-smoke, rationalized it this way: "Smokers have a distinct personality pattern. So do people who have potential for cancer. Obviously there is an overlap."

Dr. Leaf said, "That's nonsense, as far as the cancer goes. We know that it's carcinogenic. The consequences of smoking are real, it's not the personality that gives you cancer."

Then he continued: "An enzyme has been discovered, which makes some people prone to cancer if they smoke, and others are immune. The tars from the tobacco themselves are not carcinogenic, but if they are metabolized by the cells, they are converted into carcinogens, and the enzyme necessary to do this doesn't appear in all people.

"If those who have the genetic tendency will develop or increase the activity of this enzyme when they smoke, then that produces the carcinogen out of the tar. That makes it pretty clear that it isn't just your personality."

Dr. Leaf explained that, "Someone took a large group of smokers, who had been smoking for 25 years or more, and they looked at those who had developed cancer and those who didn't and the ones who had cancer had this enzyme in an active form—whereas it wasn't detected in the others. That to me is a very important discovery because it ought to alert everybody who smokes—and they ought to find out whether they're cancer-prone or not." Again, he stressed, "It's not personality. . . .

"And smoking has other effects besides producing cancer, it also has an effect on the heart and on the lungs, such as common obstructive pulmonary diseases, which are a fatal form of lung disease. It can cause emphysema. So even though cancer doesn't catch up with you, other disasters can."

Dr. Busse of Duke University said he could not speak about the effect of smoking on *viejos* in faraway places. But he quickly added "In our society, nobody comes up with any other evidence than that it's dangerous for your health."

The gerontologist Dr. Shock said that based on their Baltimore studies, those who do not smoke, particularly cigarettes, in general are apt to have longer lives than the smokers.

A doctor who devised a health and exercise program for the United States Air Force, Dr. Kenneth H. Cooper, has come down hardest on the dangers of cigarettes. He believes there is probably no such thing as a basically healthy smoker. "Even if lung cancer and other smoking-related diseases have yet to catch up with you, you are partially disabled as soon as you smoke your first pack," Dr. Cooper said. "Smoking has been called slow suicide.

"Your physical performance is affected when you smoke because the body loses some of its ability to transport oxygen from the lungs to the muscles. Carbon monoxide in cigarette smoke is a potent poison that rapidly enters the blood, combines with the hemoglobin in the red blood corpuscles and renders many of them incapable of carrying oxygen.

"The lung capacity of habitual smokers gradually shrinks, the membranes of their air passages thicken and become less efficient in gas exchange. Moreover, the cilia (tiny hairlike structures acting as brooms to sweep out the windpipe and the bronchial tubes) become paralyzed by cigarette smoking. Without this natural defense, the lungs are vulnerable to airborne intruders, dust particles and other pollutants."

I came away from the Sacred Valley aware that the *viejos* knew none of the statistics that Doctors Cooper, Shock, Busse or Leaf might quote, but rath-

that they instinctively knew and had in most cases always practiced what the wisest of philosophers all through history have always known: moderation in all aspects of living is the best rule.

8

Love—at Any Age

Strong personalities are said to be linked to the libido, to a person's sexuality. In Darwin's concept of survival of the fittest, reproductive capability played a central role.

Dr. Alex Comfort, a British scientist who has made significant contributions to gerontology, particularly to the biology of aging, has pointed out that over the centuries the hope of delaying aging has been focused on the continuation of sexual vigor and reproductive capacity. Dr. Comfort reviewed a number of rejuvenation efforts, one called gerocomy, an old man's effort to absorb virtue and youth from a young woman. This idea has permeated many societies. King David in the Old Testament practiced it. There is evidence also that the Romans held similar views. Further, as Dr. Comfort reported, this concept has some support from the modern experimental laboratory. Aged male rats will respond favorably when a young female rat is placed among them. Her presence and activities greatly improve their condition and promote their survival.

I knew, from personal experience, that all of the Old Men in Vilcabamba continued to see themselves as virile men, still living with their desires, their active libidos. Dr. Avila said he found in talking with the Old Men about their sex lives, "They still think on it, dream of it. They never get so old that they don't dream of a woman."

Sexuality, Dr. Avila added, is "a motor in human beings—it concerns one's total physiologic functioning."

Dr. Leaf also concluded that "interest in the opposite sex persists" among the *viejos* throughout their lives, and he added that such interest "is popularly regarded as the *sine qua non* of vigor and vitality. Although the ovaries of women do age and stop functioning at the menopause, usually in the late forties or early fifties, this has little effect on libido. In the male, too, aging is associated with a gradual decrease in the number of cells in the reproductive organs." Still, Dr. Leaf observed, "sexual potency in the male may persist to advanced old age." He noted that each year in America there are some 35,000 marriages of persons above age 64, and that "sex as well as companionship and economics are given as reasons."

Dr. Leaf wrote that he had asked the Old People in the Caucasus to define the age limit of "youth." Gabriel Chapnian of Gulripshi, age 117, gave a typical response: "Youth normally extends up to the age of 80. I was still young then." Professor G. E. Pitzkhelauri, head of the gerontological center in Tbilisi, Georgia, compiled data relating marital status to longevity. "He found from studies of 15,000 people older than 80 that, with rare exceptions, only the married ones attain extreme age," Dr. Leaf recalled. "Many elderly couples had been married 70, 80 or even 100 years. He concludes that marriage and a regular, prolonged sex life are very important to longevity."

In the three regions of longevity he visited, Dr. Leaf said "I saw couples who had been married for 80 years or more. Where only one of the partners survives, remarriage even at ages up to 100 are common." He concluded that people in all three areas "believe in long, happy marriages and in remarriage soon after the death of a spouse."

The quest for sexuality and fulfillment was a never-ending one among the *viejos* of Vilcabamba.

None were so old that they didn't enjoy talking about a man's need for a woman and a woman's need for a man. Desire was not dead, nor was it something that they would bury within themselves, a secret that they would not share. They loved to deal with their sexuality the way a pianist might like to use all the keys of his instrument. They enjoyed the experience of touching, of talking, of taking old affairs out in the open and examining them, as two old women with their laces. The old fragrances were, for them, still in the air. They literally used all of their senses, all of their being to express an *amor*, to preserve the illusion of the person one might have been when the ability to give seemed all of life.

Whenever I asked any *viejo* for a definition of love, he had a ready answer. It was as if he had been thinking on that very subject for the past century, perfecting his reply. And it was always marvelously simple, such as, "Love is to care for someone, *el quererse*."

Erazo represents the best example I know of a *viejo* who continued to view himself as a virile man, *muy hombre*, with a libido that was, as Dr. Avila had phrased it, a real "motor" in his life.

I well recall my first meeting with Erazo. I had borrowed a horse from Señor Toledo in the village and had set out alone for Yangana in the mountains south of Vilcabamba. I travelled over hazardous trails and at one point the path was too steep for the horse, whose own age was probably twenty years, a *viejo* as horses go. I had to dismount and lead the horse up the trail for more than an hour. The journey was one of utter isolation for me and the horse for most of the way. At one point, I came to a river and the horse, with me astride, coaxing it with my heels, swam across.

After three hours, I got to the *casa* of the *viejo*, Erazo, and dismounting, stood at a gate. A son, also named Gabriel Erazo, hurried up a sharp incline to greet me. With no words but a nod of welcome, the son, who, I saw, was blind in one eye, quickly lifted two top rungs of a log fence, and taking the bridle reins from my hands he led the horse onto his premises, and I followed.

I spoke words of gratitude for his hospitality, but soon realized he was not hearing me. He was not only partially blind but partially deaf as well. The son, with little interest in talk he could not hear, disappeared, leaving me alone with his father, who seemed eager for an exchange of thoughts. As he directed me to a bench outside the *casa* on a dirt porch under the roof's overhang, I noted that Erazo moved agilely and had sharp eyes that focused keenly on me. He obviously saw much better than I, as he wore no glasses. Talking with Erazo, I did not need to raise my voice one decibel. Moreover, he quickly grasped not *words* so much as my entire meaning.

Erazo talked to me of his long life, and his late wife, whom he met when she was a young virgin. Her name was Julia Narvaez. His eyes looked far into the distance, as if he were seeing contours of magical mountains and peaceful rivers, all that we dream as eternity. More likely, I thought, he was seeing again the contours of her buttocks, her breasts.

Erazo recalled "The priest wanted me to get married. No, *cura*, I said, if you marry such a girl you have to give beautiful dresses and good meals. But the *cura* replied, Oh no, my son, she's from a poor family, too. If you marry her, she will adapt herself to the food you give her."

The priest loaned him money, and the wedding took place. Recalling his wedding night, Erazo whispered his delight in the sensuous as well as the tender emotions she had evoked in him. She had allowed him to taste his manhood, she allowed him, with her virginity, to make him *muy macho*. "I was her first man, *el primer hombre que la uso fui yo*." With her,

he had four children. She died thirty years ago.
Erazo did not remember the year of her death, only
that at the time he was very old, "*bastante vieje-
cito.*"

I asked, "And after she died was he with another
woman?"

"No, no one, *ni mas.*"

But, Erazo insisted, he still had his desires for a
woman.

Erazo was a poet, I discovered, after I had asked,
"And what is love?" His reply came out in an al-
literative rhyme, almost a natural flowing from his
spirit:

> *El quererse es muy bonito*
> > *un hombre con una mujercita*
> *Que sea alajita*
> > *querese es bonito.*

I knew that as he talked he was saying that love
is to care for someone, that a beautiful woman is like
"a jewel." I translated his poem like this:

> To love each other is beautiful
> A man and a little woman
> She'll be like a little jewel
> To love each other is beautiful.

I asked Erazo, What is the best thing in life? And
he replied, quite simply, that *la mejor cosa* was "lying
with a woman."

I had touched on a subject that was Erazo's favorite. "If a beautiful woman is available, I can sleep
with her in the night, *como no poder dormir con ella
de noche.*"

After my initial visit to the Erazo hut in the mountains, several weeks passed, and Erazo and other
viejos who lived in mountain huts were brought to
town, to be available for examinations over a period
of several days by the visiting American and Ecuadorian doctors.

I often held Erazo's hand while the doctors were
taking their blood or skin or saliva samples, and in

between his medical examinations Erazo and I walked
in the small central square, or sat on the concrete
steps of the church, like two youngsters might, talking about life, groping for answers to ancient mysteries in life.

It was during the week that Erazo was housed in
Vilcabamba and we saw each other daily that I came
to know: *he wants to make love with me.* I knew
it before he told me, but when he told me, I did not
know what it meant, exactly.

I asked Erazo directly, What could he, at his age,
do with a woman anyway? I was attempting to force
him into saying, I *can* have an erection. Or I *can't* have
an erection. And this was what I had claimed, at least
what I had wanted to believe, was not at all important to me.

To my former husband and other men in my life,
I have said, "What is important is a tenderness, a
touching with the softness of words, or the softness
of fingertips. Art, after all, is restraint." But all of this
was in the past. I could not say any of these words
to Erazo, I could not even *think* them. I actually saw
him as most people see the aging old "fool" who
thinks he has the right to love. He is in our minds a
"dirty old man."

If a man half Erazo's age had made a proposition,
I would not have had derisive thoughts. But what
can you do? If I really had wanted tenderness and a
touching with words, with fingertips, the thoughts
would never have occurred to me to ask for an advance reading on a man's proposed performance. I
would presume, quite logically, quite normally, that a
young man was interested in sex. I would not in my
mind think of him as a "dirty young man," with an
unnatural interest in sex, as I was now prone to think
of Erazo.

But if I were capable of thinking bad thoughts of
him, Erazo apparently could see me only as a "rare
jewel," and one that he must handle delicately. I
asked what *could* he do, and he understood my query
as what *would* he do? He saw me as the typical shy

female, almost persuaded but still in need of reas-
surances that whatever he would do he would not
cause a scandal in the village, or disgrace me.

I would, he said soothingly, be safe in his hands.
"You won't become pregnant. I know a *remedio*."

The birth control remedy, he said, was made from
a plant *madre seca*. He said he would get bulbs from
the plant, dry them, wash them, pound them, make
a tea, and that if I drank that with sugar and lemon,
"nothing will happen." Then Erazo added that during the sexual act itself the woman and man must
interrupt their pleasures while she rubbed a solution
from the *madre seca* plant on the balls of her feet
and the crown of her head.

I could understand that the tea might conceivably
prevent pregnancies, and I knew from life among the
Navajo that herbal teas were used as birth control
measures. But Erazo's demonstration of rubbing a
madre seca solution on the top of his head and the
bottom of his feet was sheer mummery. But then, I
speculated I might have misunderstood his instruc-
tions. Would he run through them once more? Again,
he demonstrated as before, adding it was a good idea
to dip a comb into the *madre seca* solution "and
comb your hair, just as you comb it in the morning."
Perhaps, I thought, that would put it in your head not
to get pregnant. I was so enthralled with his instruc-
tions that I had forgotten that at my age I didn't
need to worry about it anyway. Erazo at 132 obviously thought he should.

One day I was standing by the doctors, when Erazo
marched up to the group and said to Dr. Erbe, "I
need money, *plata*, to ride the bus back home." Dick
Erbe handed him a ten *sucre* note (40 cents) and
Erazo pocketed it. I had felt slightly embarrassed
that Erazo would have stooped to ask for a handout
like that, except, as I had seen, Erazo had not
stooped. Erazo seemed sure, within himself, that the
doctors owed him that, and more.

I followed Erazo outside, and he and I sat on the
church steps, happy, as always in each others' pres-

ence. Erazo had been housed that week in an upstairs room of a two-story building and the thought crossed my mind that it might be a place where men could secure women for sex, *mujeres libres*. I asked Erazo, "Were there prostitutes in Vilcabamba?"

He said, "Yes."

"What was the price?"

He said, "Ten *sucres*."

Then patting his side where he had pocketed Erbe's ten *sucres*, he laughed gaily, "And I've got the money to pay for it."

"Had he, during the week, been with a woman?" I asked.

"No," he said, he sought a special woman who would arouse him, "*me convide la cosita*."

He had used a beautiful Castillian word, *convide*, from the verb *convidar*, so that he meant he sought a woman who would invite—and incite—him to make love to her.

After the doctors left, and Erazo had returned to his home in Communidades, I again went to visit him, travelling this time by bus. An hour and a half out from Vilcabamba, the bus reached the Mayananca river. Torrential rains had caused the stream to rise and its waters rushed furiously, breaking over huge boulders. The chauffeur of the antiquated bus, a collection of parts meticulously pieced together, decided we'd never make it across. So we sat there.

One of the passengers stripped down to his jockey shorts and swam across. He walked to a distant farm, where he borrowed two horses. He returned to the river, swam across astride one horse, leading the second. He then placed his wife and three-month-old baby on one horse and delivered them across. And then he came back for me, and helped me across. The other passengers waited on the bus for the waters to subside.

The young man and his family were going in the opposite direction from mine, so we waved goodbye. I walked for an hour and a half before I reached the *casa* of Erazo. He was sitting out under the thatched

roof overhang, on the bench, as if he were waiting for me. I embraced him, and noticed, when I sat
beside him, that he had two oranges at his side.

As he peeled oranges for me we talked. "Where are
your companions?" he asked, referring to the doctors.
"They left you alone, *sola?*" This was the aspect of my
life he could not comprehend. He tried to visualize
my life, and he questioned me. "How many days and
nights does it take to get to your country?"

I told him, "You could get there in one day."

"*Que tal!*" and again, "*Caramba!*"

The bus from Loja, I said, took five hours to get
to his house but he could get from Ecuador to the
United States in that time. I added, "You could eat
breakfast in Quito and dinner in my home in Washington, D.C."

Again he saw me alone: "You are not afraid?"

"No," I told him, adding, I was like him—not
afraid.

Then I asked, Would he like to fly to the United
States with me?

"Yes," he said. "I wouldn't be afraid."

His ability to live unafraid, his expansive personality, were traits beyond question, as inexplicable yet
natural as the wind. Erazo's personality manifest itself in his eagerness, in his laughter, and his desire
to pretend that life had just begun.

While I chatted with Erazo, a son-in-law, Flavio
Castille, who is married to Erazo's daughter, Defilia,
arrived at the mud hut, having travelled from Loja by
jeep that had managed to cross the swollen river.
Defilia, he explained, was sick, and couldn't come.
He told me that either he or she came about once a
week to help Erazo and his son look after their
property. Flavio Castille would be spending the night
in the hut, and I vaguely wondered where we would
all sleep.

While we talked, a neighbor woman, pregnant,
came to prepare our simple supper that consisted of
rice and eggs. I learned from Erazo that the pregnant
woman was a daughter of Erazo's son Gabriel.

That evening old Erazo and I went for a walk in the lovely part of the evening, and again Erazo spoke of his desires for me:

"Listen I'm pleading to you, I'm begging you, don't be selfish, don't be mean, be close with me.

"With you," Erazo continued, "I'm happy."

As he talked, he was living a most vivid life. With his desire he was himself again. He was still in a very real sense attached to the erotic world he built up in his youth and maturity.

Just as some men devote a lifetime to building up vast companies and monetary holdings so Erazo had devoted a lifetime to his romantic illusions. Erazo in a real sense *was* his dreams, his illusions.

Perhaps I should have said, No, no, enough of your words, your foolishness. But I listened. Like countless others, I hunger for praise.

Erazo's words telling me I was young, *joven*, and beautiful, *bonita*, that I aroused him to new life, new *vida*, were melting my heart, so that I soon felt like butter over an open flame, bubbly and warm.

Erazo repeated he had not been with any woman since his wife died. Then again he insisted, "I have not lost my desires. I have them—*to be with you.*"

"But there are many other women," I suggested.

"They have husbands or sweethearts, *dueños.*"

Seeing me alone, Erazo desired to protect me, to "possess" me. This was built into him, eons ago, and he found his desire for *mujer* as natural as his hunger for food.

We returned to the *casa* and, after our supper, he and I sat on the porch. He continued his amorous recitations, saying, He could touch me, woman; I could touch him, man.

". . . to touch, this is beautiful."

"What," I asked, "is it that a man likes best about a woman?"

"The woman's secret place, *la cosita.*"

"More than her intelligence, her spirit?"

"Yes, more, *si, mas!*" Then he added: "Of course there are differences. There are some who have more to offer. Now, I have desires, *deseos*. Because I find you desirable."

While Erazo and I sat on the bench outside the hut, the son Gabriel and the son-in-law Flavio Castille had cleaned the dishes. Erazo and I talked softly in order that our "secrets" would not be overheard.

To Erazo, I shook my head in a negative way. "No," I said, pleading with him, "don't do this."

I was going into the hut to be sleeping in one room with three men and one, the Old Man, wanted me in the way a man wants a woman, and I was looking down to his dirty crusty feet, knowing that he probably had not been in a bathtub in all of his life.

Darkness came and Erazo and I went inside the hut whose ceiling was about as high as I am tall—not much more than five feet. It was smaller than a small child's bedroom. There were no beds, as such, merely boards along sides of the adobe walls. Flavio Castille showed me the board-beds where Erazo and his son would sleep and the board-bed where I would sleep. I would almost be touching distance from Erazo. The three board-beds consumed all the living-sleeping space, and Flavio Castille said he would sleep right above me, up on bamboo rafters—in the attic, as it were. There were four or five rickety stairsteps to get there. I volunteered I would sleep in the loft and started climbing the rickety steps, but Flavio Castille moved me aside and climbed the steps himself.

In the night, I lay down on the board-bed that was covered by one blanket, like a hard, rough, thin saddle blanket, and I had another blanket over me. I felt half paralyzed with anxiety. My thoughts ran rampant: Is he coming here? I attempted to relax, to let my mind lie fallow. I was cold, nervous. My fears were ravelled knots.

Small night creatures gorged themselves on my flesh. I tried to distinguish fleas from bed bugs. I tried praying.

I tried to remember all the thoughts and phrases that I used to get through the nights when I was ill.

And I wanted to think pure thoughts: What was my happiest time? My happiest time *was*—my happiest time was not in the past; *it is yet to be!*

I am aware of his stirring. Is he coming to me? No, he is passing water in a bedside pot. My board creaks with every move that I make, just as his bed broadcasts his movements.

I try to convince myself it is amusing—my being dominated by a man who says he is 132! Also, I worry not so much about what might happen, but that it can happen with two other men in the same hut. I fear they will see me unclean, immoral—corrupting the morals of an old man.

Erazo coughs. I feel the dampness, the cold, hard bed. I listen to a distant Mayananca river as it rushes over its rocks.

I check my watch. It is midnight.

I try to reassure myself, and again attempt to be amused by the "facts" of a strong-bodied, strong-willed woman being frightened by an old, very old man. Why does Erazo frighten me? I know. It is because I now see him as a *dirty old* man.

The Old Man moves out of his bed. I feel certain, in the darkness, he is moving toward my bed. The son Gabriel shouts, "Where are you going, *Donde vas?*"

And the father says, "I'm not going anywhere, *no estoy saliendo.*"

And again, the quietness.

I am experiencing sexuality and life in the raw, and I see that they are the same: terrifying, awesome, overpowering, dreadful but desirable.

I curl up into the womb position, trying to keep warm.

Later, there is a stirring.

"Gabriel!" the old father shouts to his half-deaf son. "Gabriel!" The son, now dead asleep, does not respond. Erazo again shouts and gets no response.

"Gabriel, don't you have a match to light a candle?"

The son stirs and lights a candle and there is a flicker of light in the windowless hut.

The Old Man wants to talk, but the son does not hear. I hold my body motionless, my eyes shut. "There is nothing," old Erazo says. And again he repeats the phrase, "There is nothing" with great fury. What is he missing? Is he looking for a possession and not finding it? Is this some sort of philosophic summation of his long life?

There is no way that I can understand the meaning of his words. Perhaps, even, he is talking in his sleep. I cannot know.

Morning eventually comes, and I get up at the first light. Gabriel runs to pick oranges for me to take on the bus. Erazo looks sad at my leaving, and says "I'm praying that it does not rain on you. It is not a happy time to travel *wet*." He is expressing his concern for me, his love for me.

He then walked down the road with me to await the bus to Vilcabamba. And when I boarded the bus, we waved goodbye. I find a seat and I listen to the passengers talk of the aged Erazo. One said, "He must be 100." Another, a very old man, said, "No, older. He was an *old* man when I was a child."

As we moved away, I saw that the eyes of Erazo were alert, they were filled with his concern for me, they were searching for me—among the passengers on the bus.

9

A Mixing of Generations—
And a Respect for the Elderly

The *viejos* live in close-knit families with all of the psychological cushions and spiritual comforts that a sharing of life with loved ones provides. Although they live on dirt floors in primitive huts fashioned out of mud and sticks, they have an "at home" sense of security that somehow seems missing in our more abundant society, where few Americans live where they were born and where a universal skepticism has diluted the homely virtues by which we once lived. We have to a large extent cut ourselves from our moorings, and change, almost too rapid to comprehend, keeps robbing us of our sense of place.

The *viejos* are never adrift. They are "in place" at birth, most die where they were born, and throughout their long lives they are rooted to loved ones, friends and relatives, who provide them with a secure psychological haven, a barricade against the strangeness, the aloneness, of most other people. The Ecuadorian doctor, Guillermo Vela, put it simply: "In Vilcabamba, the *viejos* are never alone. I believe this is fundamental, primordial."

In Vilcabamba, one begins to know himself from his earliest childhood by standing inside a circle of love and protection, looking outward, aware that he is vulnerable and dependent on others. All his life the *viejo* has known that he can never be an isle unto himself, a sovereign, separate entity, beholden to no man, no woman, no child. He builds a strength by recognizing a weakness, a need for family. He makes a ritual out of his needs. A man will say to a woman, or a woman will tell a man, "You are my life, *mi vida*. I depend on you. I need you."

Phrases that give strength and reassurance to persons of any age are especially tonic to the elders. Sons, daughters, grandchildren constantly reaffirm their need of them, by word, gesture and deed. The verbal essence of this deep avowal of affection and respect for the aged can be summed up: "You are the reason why we are here. You are first in the family. We need your superior wisdom, we need your wise judgments, we learn from you." And the *viejos* respond, with their alert minds and their useful hands. The clearest lesson here is that an elderly man or woman, like the rest of us, often tends to become what others perceive him or her to be.

I never saw a *viejo* patronized by his juniors or treated with a false deference. The Vilcabamba elderly are presumed to be wise and rational. I saw no case of senility among them, no evidence of dotage, no forlorn sense of uselessness. In the United States, age is a measure of declining utility. Mandatory retirement provisions consign able, hearty, willing men and women to idle lives, and the collective conscience is assuaged by the thought that they are being rewarded for a lifetime of honorable toil.

We have been oriented to a social system that demands productivity and beats the drum endlessly for consumption. Unlike the young, the old do not have a place of honor in the statistics of consumption. The increase of our old has created what one expert has called a new type of "racial problem," discrimination, neglect and disdain. Our old people are often devalued, unloved. We love children better and take more interest in them. By emphasizing youth and putting our old people away in institutions, we have in effect been saying that "we"—the young and the middle aged—will never become "them." Such a separation does not occur in Vilcabamba, however, because of the mixing of the generations.

I often reflected on the needs that the old and the young have for each other as I sat on a bench outside a stucco house with Angel Modesto, mentioned earlier as the man who said he had smoked thirty to forty cigarettes a day since he was eighteen. His great-grandson, Luis Fernando, not yet two, usually was at his side. They seemed sewn from the same bolt of cloth. They walked at the same pace, with the gait of kinship. They had time and love and attention for each other. They seemed to exist in each other's eyes, in the awareness of one for the other. For long stretches, I would watch the tireless Luis Fernando romping and running and laughing, testing his legs and his arms and his place in the world, and daily growing more secure in the knowledge that the loving eyes of his great-grandfather countenanced with enormous approbation his every move. Each was aware of the other and shared their love with an unaffected ease. I felt having his great-grandfather, whom he called "Little Daddy," *Papito,* in his life was as important for Luis Fernando's sense of well-being, now and in his future, as his having nursed from his mother's breast.

Once I said to Modesto: "Come to the central plaza and let me take your picture."

Since there was so little to do in the village, Modesto readily agreed to the small adventure. He took Luis Fernando by the hand and the three of us strolled along the dirt road to the central plaza. Modesto decided to have his hair cut, and I took photos of him seated in the one-chair barber shop, with his great-grandson on his lap.

The relationship between grandchildren and grandparents in many primitive communities has been strong, as marginal members of the community were freed from the serious life of the adults. One good example are the Navajo young and old who share close relationships. Many of their tribal leaders have recalled that as children they lived with their grandparents, who were considered the custodians of knowledge. A respected Navajo leader, Peterson Zah, said when he was a boy his grandfather waked him in the predawn hours "and we ran races over the mountains." The grandfather wanted the boy strong in body and spirit.

When most American people lived on farms in the country there were tasks for all members of the family, grandparents included. They were needed for many chores. With the move to the big cities and a change of lifestyle and pace, with so many of us living in small apartments rather than rambling farmhouses, the influence of the grandparents has declined, and everyone has been a loser, the children, the grandparents and society in general.

Many gerontologists say longevity is directly and significantly related to the degree of modernization, with the status of the aged high in primitive societies and lower in modern societies. Donald Cowgill in his book *Aging and Modernization* wrote that "In primitive societies, older people tend to hold positions of political and economic power, but in modern societies such power is possessed by only a few." He added that "the individualistic value system of western society tends to reduce the security and status of older people."

When parents in the United States grow old, they often move out of their homes and live with their children, but in Vilcabamba, grown children often return to live with their parents. Rosalie, daughter of Gabriel Sanchez and Maria Petrona Yunga, had children outside of wedlock and she and her children lived with her aged parents. And Dolores and her children lived with her parents, Manuel Ramon and Barbarita Ocampo. A nephew, 21, lived with his aunt, Micaela Quezada, who has lived in the same house for 40 years. A daughter Rosa and her son lived with her mother, Señora Mariana Toledo. The old mother often walked to a nearby *hacienda* to labor in the field. "But I always return home at night," she told me. "I want to sleep in my own bed. I have many friends among the *campesinos,* and they beg me to stay with them, especially when it is raining, but I always return home."

In the evenings when Señora Toledo and her daughter Rosa and I visited, we were three females crowded around a small table, made for two, and Rosa's son, not finding space to sit in the small mud-and-sticks hut, disappeared into dark corners. We had only a small candle on the table for light. The intimacy made us one family, and in this closeness and simplicity I felt a deep spiritual affinity for both the aged mother and her daughter. Señora Toledo, who lost seven of her fourteen children in childbirth, was accustomed to large gatherings of people, and she always took a maternal interest in me, begging me to stay with them more often. As she put it: "Often it is just the three of us, and you make it more like family."

Rosa never forgot that her mother was head of the household, and there was no hint of suppressed rebelliousness or resentment. In other homes that I visited, the children and grandchildren looked to their elders for wise counsel, for knowledge and judgments and final decisions. In the Erazo hut, for instance, when I asked the son, Gabriel, a *viejo* himself, for a weather forecast, or any opinion, such as the best method of raising corn or the best remedy for an illness, he would respectfully defer to Erazo senior: "*Mi padre* knows better than I."

In their setting, the old father represented a storehouse of knowledge. He was the keeper of the wisdom. He knew the soil, the water, the trees, the herbs, and because of his longer years and wider experience, he was the teacher, the son still the pupil.

A priest, who had found no help from medical authorities in Loja, came to Erazo with leprosy, *una lepra.* And Erazo said, "I can tell you a simple cure." Erazo went into the mountains and brought back an ample supply of the plant *matico,* and made his remedy: "You put leaves in water and boil. Afterwards save the leaves, dry them, crumble them into powder and apply on the sores." After the priest had applied the *matico* remedy three times a day for 15 days, "The sores disappeared." Erazo said *matico* was good for cuts, burns, bruises, open sores. Erazo knew a plant *guayuza* "that will make a woman fertile," and a plant *madre seca* "that will prevent a pregnancy," and another plant *chine,* "good for rheumatism," and *escausel,* "to prevent bruises." *Nogal,* he said, "was good for your blood." Erazo knew where to find the best *alditamo,* "It grows high in the mountains, has very fine leaves that look like needles. It is good for the bones in your body, especially for the cheek bones in your face and for eyesight, for vision."

The wisdom that Erazo had gleaned over his long years was put into practice every day of his life, and he would, for as long as he lived, be in a position of authority, enjoying the respect of his son and others in his family. This position of authority within the family, psychologists have stressed, adds strength to an older person, enables him to live more happily, and to stretch out his years in usefulness.

The term *elder* has, in fact, commonly denoted prestige, honor, an esteemed designation for a headman or councilman. And throughout history, aged men have served their people as headmen, and chieftains. Moses held the leadership of the Israelites to a very great age and until his death. Among the Navajo, old men become the most respected doctors and priests or medicine men, entrusted to exorcise spirits, work charms and treat disease. Most tribes, anthropologists and sociologists indicate, have had old men as chiefs, councilmen and advisors.

Dr. Vela commented on this, observing that "In Vilcabamba the old person continues to be head of the family. He is a respected person. In Quito, also, the old person is practically the center of the family. Others respect him, and are considerate of him. In Vilcabamba the *viejo* participates in the life, others consult him, for his opinions, ideas. He still has personality to give his judgments and he knows that his opinions will be respected. This is a factor that influences his life."

Dr. Leaf said that in his studies of the very old in Ecuador, Russia and Hunza he had found a striking feature common to all three cultures—the high status of the aged. "Each of the very elderly persons I saw lived with family and close relatives—often an extensive household—and occupied a central and privileged position within this group. The sense of family continuity is strong. There is also a sense of usefulness. Even those well over 100 for the most part continue to perform essential duties and contribute to the economy of the community. These duties included weeding in the fields, feeding the poultry, tending flocks, picking tea, washing the laundry, cleaning house, or caring for grandchildren, all on a regular basis. In addition, the aged are esteemed for the wisdom that is thought to derive from long experience, and their word in the family group is generally law."

The Boston doctor found it interesting to observe that in the areas of longevity he visited, "social status is largely age-dependent. The older a person is, the higher he or she is regarded both by contemporaries and by the young. I am now convinced," Dr. Leaf continued, "that when the social environment encourages one to feel socially useful and needed in the economy, and to be looked up to and revered as a wise figure, the extremely elderly keep their mental faculties and physical abilities so that they can respond appropriately. This is quite contrary to prevailing trends in modern industrialized societies, which tend to emphasize youth and to regard old people as useless and standing in the way of progress."

Living among people such as Señora Toledo and Señor Sanchez, and Señor Erazo, I learned that it is not a bank account that can give an old person a sense of security so much as the assurance that he or she never will live alone, nor die alone. Regardless of his age in the Sacred Valley the *viejo* never feared being abandoned, or being put away in an institution, unwanted, neglected, left to wither and die.

In nursing homes in this country, where old people are hidden and forgotten—except for occasional visits by a son or daughter, between rounds of golf or marketing—the elderly often lose their sense of reality. The "reality" of being old in Vilcabamba, where one is respected and always "at home," is different from the "reality" of being abandoned and adrift and left to expire in an institution.

In the United States a person can work hard all of his or her life, only to reach the heap of obsolescence. The reality is that the old in this country have every right to feel "depressed." A *viejo*, such as Manuel Ramon, will never know that kind of desolation, that kind of abandonment and depression.

Once a doctor in the course of his routine questioning asked Ramon, "Are you often depressed?"

Ramon replied quite simply, "Only if I have a reason to be." As an example, he recalled that "Once my home was burned to the ground, and I was depressed." But he built it back again and felt happy to be alive. It would never have occurred to Ramon to think of "depressed" and "very old" as synonymous.

10

Dealing with Stress

In many tests of old people in the United States the doctors found that a person's "mental attitude" was a key, often listed as the most important one, for his or her long life. Not exercise, not diet, but how one viewed himself, his acceptance of self and his own idea of "life satisfaction."

A unique study, thought to be the longest continuous analysis of its type in the country, suggests that our emotional makeup may reveal our susceptibility to cancer, coronaries, mental ills and suicide. Under Dr. Caroline Bedell Thomas, Professor Emeritus of Medicine at Johns Hopkins University, certain details in the profile of an individual (starting as early as perhaps only 20) are being found to foreshadow the likelihood of disease or death overtaking him or her prematurely. Dr. Thomas, who has conducted her studies over a period of 28 years, commented that "We all know race horses don't pull plows and plow horses don't win races," but she added, perhaps we don't realize how people are also limited by their personalities, "and that when these limits are ignored severe illness may result."

She has made extensive studies on what she terms *habits of nervous tension* and she learned that how a person responds to stress determines subsequent illness. It may not be the stress in one's life that is all important, then, but one's ability or inability to deal with stress.

Unlike those whose fortunes are outraged by a thousand wounds, and who withdraw from life to lick them, the Vilcabamba natives lead lives that are open, receptive, *vulnerable*. If they have built armor against hurt, it is nowhere displayed. Like innocent animals of the field, they seek no shelter from the thrusts and cuts of everyday living. They seem to recognize a maxim of their spiritual guides that "only the gods go woundless on their way." Together with that most Spanish of philosophers, Unamuno, they know it is natural to dislike grief, but totally unnatural to attempt to deny grief, when grieving and loving are the emotional grist of living itself.

The peace and tranquility that one found in the lives of the people might mean that the *viejos* had no tensions or stresses in their lives, or that they had learned how to deal with them. Dr. Hans Selye, a Canadian researcher, has called stress, and how we deal with it, a key factor to longevity. In his original research on the dangers of stress in the aging process, Dr. Selye had pinpointed it as the villain. He had held a "watchspring theory," that the human body supposedly is wound up and set for a certain length of time. And that each stress situation draws upon our reserve of adaptation energy, with aging coming on when the reserve begins to develop serious deficits.

To me, the *viejos* seemed fashioned out of a recipe that Selye had written. I went to visit them because I had heard they were old. But I stayed with them because they were themselves, a most lovable people, from whom I wanted to learn. Each one seemed to believe that he would become all that he had given away.

I never before experienced a people who had so little and gave so much. Without any material possessions, they somehow assert their personalities, their individuality, their right to be giving. Of all the Biblical injunctions they had heard from the Spanish priests, the *viejos* seem to have taken "It is more blessed to give, than to receive" as their maxim in life.

A *viejo* such as Señor Sanchez, oppressed by the *hacienda* system, seemed to have had two choices: to hate or to grow more compassionate. And having "nothing" he wanted to give even that away. As one example: I was leaving their primitive hut and Sanchez and Maria Petrona Yunga followed me a few steps down the rocky path, toward the village—followed me with the tenderness in their eyes I have seen in my own mother, and then Maria Petrona as a token of her affection put two fresh eggs in my hands. She was in her own way dealing with her life of nothingness, her poverty, her "misery"—by saying I am "rich" if I think of myself that way. It was ironic that I should be the recipient of the gift. I had been the stranger, asking them to take me in. I was indebted to them. But they did not choose to see it that way. They wanted still to be giving. And they earned love and respect for themselves in this fashion.

One had to know the poverty in their lives to appreciate the fact that eggs and milk were as rare and wonderful to the *viejos* as champagne and caviar might be in the lives of the average American. The two eggs were the best that they had to give.

There were other instances when I found myself the recipient of two eggs. Once Erazo and I walked a long distance to a neighbor's hut to borrow a pail of milk. Erazo himself never drank milk, but he made the journey because he knew I liked milk in my coffee. We arrived at a primitive hut, and the señora greeted us in beautiful Castillian phrases, as if she herself were of royal lineage. All of her words meant, "Come and rest awhile, and this home is your home, *mi casa es su casa*." We chatted awhile, and she gave Erazo a pail of milk, and as we were leaving she presented me, as a token of her generosity, with two eggs.

One day I asked Leonor Cartuche, 103, to let me take her picture with her daughter Maria Cabrera, 80, and the old woman said shyly, "But I wouldn't have any money to pay you for the picture." I thought of all the countries I had visited where the natives expected you to pay them. After I explained to Señora Cartuche that she need not pay me, she posed for her picture. Later, she sent a neighbor, a small child, to the hut where I was staying with a gift: two oranges.

Living among the *viejos*, I never heard them quarrel or fight or dispute with each other. They had what I would consider a "high" culture in this regard. They spoke beautiful, elegant Castillian, with ample flourishes of tenderness. Their words themselves often were caresses.

Vilcabamba has only two policemen, and one, Hugo Gordova, 30, said he was not bothered with any real "crimes" as such. "One of the main problems is heavy drinking and rowdiness, but none of that is by the viejos—it's the young, and especially students who come here from Loja."

I asked, "And why were the young being rowdy and disturbing the peace?"

"I think it's the influence of the movies they see in Loja. They see so much violence," the policeman said.

"Well, did anyone ever die as a result of a crime in Vilcabamba?" I asked.

"Once a young man died because he fell off his horse drunk," Gordova said.

"And on another occasion a young man killed himself. He picked up a gun and thought it was not loaded, but it went off and killed him."

Once I discussed the incidence of crime with Manuel Pardo and Alberto Roa. "Did they know of a case of anyone killing another human being?"

"Yes," said Roa, and he turned to Pardo, "Don't you remember Isauro Perez at Palmira killed Ortega, for taking his wife?" And Pardo nodded, "Si, si," he did indeed recall the incident, and they discussed the aspects of the crime as graphically as if they had seen it on the TV evening news, except of course they had never seen TV in their lives.

"When was that murder?" I asked, thinking maybe it was last week.

"Oh," said Roa, "that must have been fifty years ago."

"No, more, *mas*," insisted Pardo, who said it had to have been seventy years ago.

It was the only such incident that they could remember, and it had registered sharply in each of their minds.

"Did the people keep many guns?" I asked.

"No," Pardo said. "Why would we? The people here are sane, *gente sana*."

Señor Manuel Pardo seemed a perfect illustration of a man dealing with stress in the Hans Selye way.

Señor Pardo lived a hard, sparse life, with fewer earthly goods than those who live below the poverty line in more advanced environments. But he had accumulated a special brand of gentility, free of hatred, immune to violence.

If violence breeds violence, pain breeds understanding. Manuel Pardo had had his soul seared because of his love for a woman, and when I sat down to talk with him, at the one table outside the small Pedro Alberca beer parlor, across from the town square, Pardo spoke to me of that greatest of all dramatic events: the human heart in conflict with itself.

I had gone through the usual questions with him, a slight man but strong as a steel cable, in an effort to glean a truth, as if factual data could in any sense measure a man. In any case, one has to begin somewhere.

"How old are you?" I asked.

"Ninety-six," he said. And what time did he get up in the mornings? "Sometimes five, sometimes six, when the sun comes up." And was he born in Vilcabamba? "Yes."

Pardo was twenty-five when he married Julia Cocios. They bred two sons, Efrain Pardo, who is now seventy, and Umberto, sixty-five; and two daughters, Mariana Pardo, now fifty, and Luz Aurora, forty-five. His wife Julia Cocios died in giving birth to Luz Aurora, and Pardo was left with the newborn baby and the other children to raise.

While Pardo and I talked, sharing a beer, *cerveza*, at the sidewalk table, a cluster of townspeople encircled us. They were not eavesdropping so much as participating. Some put their elbows on the table, their faces so close to mine I could count wrinkles.

Pardo, pretending I was the only person listening, told me that after Julia Cocios had died he had taken a second wife, Luz Albertina Cajas. I then asked:

How old was he when he married the second time?

"Seventy-one," he said.

"And how old was your wife?"

"Twenty," he replied.

Interrupting our dialogue, an old toothless woman leaned over our table, nearly knocking over my beer. Pointing her finger at Pardo, she cackled derisively, "Hey, Manuel, you got married to a child, *la hija*."

He smilingly, yet sadly accepted their sardonic laughter. "So it goes, *así es*," he commented.

With *"la hija"* Pardo had three sons, *barones*, Angel Manuel, Rojilla and Roque; and one daughter, Amada Cruz.

And so he'd had four children by each wife? I asked.

"Yes, I have eight children. The youngest is fourteen."

And how long had he been married to his second wife?

"Twenty-five years."

And was he still in love with this woman?

"Ah, no."

After a long silence, Pardo continued, "This woman acted bad."

With another man?

"Yes. Not just one, two, *dos hombres*."

Now it became clear why the townspeople had so freely gathered to laugh at Pardo. In almost any, latino community a man may easily kill "his" woman if she is untrue to him. An Ecuadorian once said to me he could lose all his money, his job, his home, his mother, but if "my woman were untrue, it would destroy me." Those who know, and in small villages everyone does, mock the cuckold, *cornudo*. That for a latino is the worst name in the Spanish language.

I asked Pardo, Were the two men friends of his?

"Might have been friends, but they're enemies now."

"You've seen them?"

"Yes. And because of this I've suffered. I don't do anything well. I can't continue to work hard, to advance."

"You would, with a good woman?"

"*Sí*, I could work with zest, *con ganas*. I'd have a reason for my life and work."

"How long ago did this happen with the two men?"

"Two years ago."

"You can't forget?"

"No. I can't forget."

He said he tried to keep his senses because of his daughter. He added, "I hope nothing bad happens here."

Was he in the same *casa* with his wife?

"No, the woman who can deceive you can also poison you."

He sighed, explaining, "When you love a person it's like it should never end. And when it has ended you want . . . that old love is what you most want."

"She continues to be with other men?" I asked.

"Yes, she's with other men."

Again, a silence. It was an integral part of our dialogue.

"I know very well," he continued.

Well, what could he do? I asked. Was he going to kill her, *matar*?

And he gave a little laugh, not a cheerful one, but a laugh that was close to a cry, "No, no *matar*," he said. "But I feel heavy, *harto, harto*."

In the time he was married to Luz, was he not untrue to her? Didn't he have another woman?

"No."

"You didn't ever deceive her?"

"No, not once."

How many times in his life had he been in love?

"Too many—they were in my youth. They were before I married her. But little by little you begin to restrain yourself. The years pass by and the heart wants a home."

And what is more important, sex or tenderness?

"To care, *querer*. To have a good heart. To create a tenderness, a fondness, a caring for another, this is *amor*, no? When a person acts right, then nothing wrong happens. This is what a person cares for most."

He was saying the most important thing in his life would be *if* she acted right. "Little by little, one sees what has happened in the past," he continued.

But then he abruptly interrupted his train of thought, and he was out of himself, out of his past, dropping it as easily as a woman might her shawl. Redirecting his attention to me, he asked:

"Do you like to drink milk?"

I was so taken aback by this swift hurdle of *his* past to *our* present that I muttered, "Who, me? Yo? Like milk?"

"*Le gusta tomar leche?*" He apparently construed my surprised reaction and inability to reply to his question as a desire for milk.

"*Mañana* then. Where are you staying?"

In the little *casa* of Señor Churo, I told him.

"When the milk comes in, I'll go get some for you. Don't worry about it."

I knew that, in terms of cost, his buying the milk for me was the equivalent of my giving a friend a new hi-fi set. He had worked with machete an entire day to earn enough to make this gesture. He was following his heart. His heart said giving is better than getting.

"It is necessary to do something if we care for those who come to visit us. To give life—to life," Pardo said. But more than that, he was saying that while he still wanted the Old Love in his life he knew that it was dead, and that he had to somehow go on living. And he was saying, "Help me. Let me give to you."

The next morning, Pardo, a man of his word, was out early, purchased a pitcher of warm milk and brought it to me. I was seated on a bench, outside the Churo *casa*. I accepted the gift, although I knew I was the person in Vilcabamba who probably needed the precious commodity least of all.

Sitting, holding the pitcher of milk, I thought of the persons I have known to say, "I loved, but was not loved in return." Often, one feels that this is the fault of the other person. Pardo, as poor and "miserable" as his existence on dirt floors may be, was *earning* a love. And by being a "hoarder of goodwill," he was (regardless of his awareness of the psychological implications) making his environment less stressful.

Despite his suffering, he did not barricade his heart against others. He accepted his grief, as a part of life.

Unamuno understood this "tragic sense of life." He wrote, "The satisfied, the happy, do not love; they fall asleep in habit, near neighbors to annihilation. . . . Man is the more man—that is, the more divine—the greater capacity for suffering, or rather for anguish."

One psychiatrist has defined successful aging as the ability to deal with change in nondestructive ways. I knew that Pardo could have dealt with his unfaithful wife in a destructive way. In many Latin countries infidelity is an "acceptable" reason for murder. But after telling me about his soul being seared, Pardo went to pray. I saw him that evening, on his knees, asking *Dios* to keep his heart filled with love, not hate. As he told me, "If I turn to revenge and punishment, I am the only one who is going to lose." The *viejos* were not immune to temptations, or to evil. They dealt with stress, and somehow made it "bless" their lives.

11

Coming to Terms
with Your Life

I do not want to paint a picture of an ideal place
and perfect people. The *viejos* live far from paradise.

And I realize that the average visitor to Vilcabamba
might well be appalled by the poverty of the people, the "nothingness" of their lives. The average visitor, who leaves his radio, television, telephone, automobile, hot and cold running water, electricity, gas,
central heating—all of which are missing in the lives
of the *viejos*—would no doubt see them as "simple,"
"dirty," "uneducated" peasants.

We, in our highly materialistic, pragmatic society,
put a high value on acquiring "facts"—even if they
don't add up to any truth—and also on acquiring creature comforts and *earthly* goods.

Living with the *viejos* I came to be impressed with
more profound, philosophical aspects of life, with
what we might call the *eternal* values.

A *viejo* seemed to know that growing older was
akin to growing in wisdom, understanding, tolerance,
and faith, not retrogressing or falling fallow. In a profound sense, aging implies a renewal of self, the
ceaseless quest for self-identity. To a *viejo* such as
the 110-year-old Manuel Ramon, living in the remote

simplicity of Vilcabamba, unassailed by the distractions of the teeming world outside, it was natural to view life as a whole, and realize that the big events were not written in politics or wars or money matters but in the human heart. Life in Vilcabamba was reduced, depending on one's outlook, to the "nothingness"—or the "all"—of life: living and dying. Some *viejos*, such as Manuel Ramon, took time to examine life and the examination of life gave it flavor, enriched it, made it all worthwhile.

In one respect Ramon was like an old Greek philosopher looking in on himself. He had time to review his life, to pick and choose among his recollections, to embellish the episodes he cherished, to know the color and texture and perhaps even the scent in the air of those days that were most special to him. He gave time to the study of himself, to the manner in which he related to the universe. He lived with the pleasure of the "puzzle" that life gave—the beauty that was mystery. It was, perhaps, as simple as sleeping out under the stars, trying to count them and knowing that you never could.

Once I asked Señor Ramon, "What was the happiest time in your life?"

He did not have to stop and think, as so many of my sophisticated busy friends must do, often in vain. Ramon recalled immediately going across to the other side of the mountains, *"atras de las cordilleras,"* —and he made it sound like a dream world—sleeping out and hunting bear.

Ramon spent his waking hours with the sun. When the sun rose he climbed the mountain to work in his field, and when the sun set his day ended and he went to bed. Once as we talked about his life of hard work, he paused briefly, and I reached over and felt the muscles in his arms and observed that he was very strong, *muy hombre*.

His hunger for a word of praise was plain, but he didn't make much of it. He explained with a laconic eloquence that he only wielded a *lampa* and machete on the stubbled land. And with consummate mod-

esty and grace added, "I don't do a great thing."
Tolstoy at the end of his years said as much. And Father Leclerc wrote, "When one comes to the end . . .
a man's life, it's nothing much."

Each of us makes the word "life" mean what he or
she chooses it to mean. And when Ramon said, "I
don't do a great thing," he was not saddened by his
full acceptance of reality. Indeed, he had smiled as
he summarized his life, indicating a quiet satisfaction
within himself at having come to terms with the
specific conditions of his life. Ramon had gained nothing in worldly fame, nothing the way the protagonist
Slocum in the Heller novel, *Something Happened*,
had measured his "success." Slocum gained "success" despite his fears of closed doors, and his co-
workers. He hated having a mentally deficient child,
he did not enjoy his other children and wished he
could be divorced from his wife. Ramon, on the other
hand, had found an abandoned child in the fields
(later, he learned, the child was mentally deficient)
but he had felt lucky he had still another person to
love. Ramon, in touch and at peace with his real
inner self, could accept the responsibilities of the
choices he had made. He could make commitments
to loved ones, to friends, to values and ethical standards. He was content with his occupational and
familial roles and encountered no great problems in
them. Slocum, on the other hand, regardless of a new
promotion and a bigger salary, remained discon-
tented, depressed, fear ridden.

The doctors and I often discussed the meaning of the
word "happiness" as it applied to men such as Ramon.
We knew countless rich, "successful" men who were
real persons who seemed exactly like the fictionalized
Slocum. If you met Slocum, he would want you to
know that he was not a happy man. If you met the
viejo Ramon, he would tell you that he was a happy
man. This leads one to question the general definition
of "successful." Perhaps one day we will redefine it,
admitting that in one sense if the individual thinks he
is happy, he is "successful."

Señor Ramon had never studied psychology out of a book but he would be the first to know to what a large extent his mind controls his body. And probably the most important part of biological aging may well be simply how one feels about himself.

After his round-the-world search for clues to longevity, Dr. Leaf commented on the importance of attitude, or zest for living:

"For a physician who was raised on the pathological and physiological basis of illness, I must say I have been struck increasingly, as I have looked at these problems of the aged, how much of illness comes out of psychological and emotional situations."

The *viejos* of Vilcabamba stayed flexible, not only in body but in spirit. That is, they learned long ago to cooperate with the inevitable. Old Erazo was one good example.

Like the Greek slave Epictetus who counseled men to wish for nothing that was not under their control, he refused to worry. He had relegated his big problems to *Papa Dios* and *Mama Virgen*. Once, Erazo related, when he was so ill he almost died, relatives wanted to take him to a hospital in Loja. "I said, No, maybe I would die, and they would be left with debts. I talked with *Papa Dios* and *Mama Virgen* and asked them to look for me. And to help me still, and fix it so I could get cured more easily. The next day I felt like getting up. I met some *amigos* and they gave me some yucca and potatoes and bananas, and didn't charge me. I put these in my *bultito* I carried over my shoulder, and I met a man selling a quarter of a *carcass*, and I wondered, What kind of meat is this, bear, *oso*, maybe? So I asked and the man said 'This is *carne* of burro.' I asked him to lower the price for me, and he said 'Why not?' So I took it home, and cooked it, and this *carne* made me well."

Erazo could not logically explain why he thought meat from a burro had cured his illness, but then Erazo, who had never taken an aspirin, much less gone to a doctor, was convinced, in his own mind, that it had. The perception was totally real and would tolerate no modern, sophisticated, contrary view.

Old Erazos moods were often paradoxical. One moment he would tell you quite frankly: I know that I am nothing more than a *peon*. And then, his eyes shining, like a child's, he would boast: I am really good at what I do. Erazo had an incredible storehouse of memories, and surprisingly, they usually were pleasant ones. For instance, Erazo recalled his "most pleasant" days working for a priest, Cura Bustamente, who owned a *hacienda* in Guaicapamba. "I played a guitar, and the priest danced with the pretty girls," Erazo said, smiling. The priest died of a strange malady and Erazo went to work at the Comunidades *hacienda*. "It rained for a week without stopping, and then they gave me a parcel of land, a *finca* to work for myself."

Could he remember the name of the *patron?*

"Si." And Erazo recalled the name Jose Maria Montero as easily as if he had gone to work for him yesterday.

Erazo wanted me to understand that he knew a lot about planting and cultivating. This was what made a *man* in his world, knowing the soil. His *patron* "gave me a very good position," Erazo said proudly. I felt he longed to exist in my eyes, in my approval of the good work he had done, as another man might show me his medals or his newspaper clippings.

All of his life Erazo had done nothing but work with his hands, in the fields, with a machete and with the crude handmade hoe or *lampa*, and regardless of how the *patron* might have praised him, Erazo was forever the *campesino*, the *peon*, and yet he looked back on his work with the pride of a tutored professional man, seeing nothing menial or demeaning about it. It was, he repeated, "A good position." He obviously was one of those eternal optimists who could get more out of a situation than was really there. And walking proof that it's not what happens to you that counts but how you take it.

Erazo had a childlike guilelessness, an openness. He never felt threatened by my knocking on the inner recesses of his psyche, asking what to another might seem a rude or impertinent question. Erazo always assumed I meant well.

It was this openness, this total acceptance, of himself, of me, of those conditions around us, that most impressed me. He simply wanted you to know that we could talk as frankly as if there were no secrets between us. With me, he was saying, there are no locked compartments, nothing that you can't know. He seemed a striking exception to the general theory that when the average man grows very old, he grows more suspicious, more turned in on himself.

Erazo always was like a teenager, who with a friend is exploring the world of self-discovery. Subjects might range from the sublime to the clinical. And on one occasion—previous to my staying the night in his hut—it included an inquiry I made about his prostate gland. I had become interested in this subject since the prostate seems to be the overall controller of a man's sexual health. And sexual health is intimately connected with a man's vigor, and physical and mental general well-being.

My inquiry began in his garden at Comunidades. He had shown me trees and plants which seemed to have sprouted up and produced without any planning. Erazo stopped and plucked an orange, and peeled sections of it, handing them to me. He pointed out papayas growing next to avocados that fought for their survival among banana trees. A few coffee plants were mixed with tobacco plants.

Eventually we sat down for a rest, along the banks of the Mayananca river, which sped playfully over rocks in front of us. Now I determined to learn more about Señor Erazo's urinary habits. In the United States, one out of three men is said to suffer prostatic enlargement, but none of the doctors who had gone to Vilcabamba had ever investigated the subject among the *viejos*, so I decided to be straightforward and blunt.

"Señor Erazo," I asked, "how often do you have to pass water, *agua*?" He smiled and continued to gaze at the stream in front of us. Perhaps I was using the wrong word for urinate.

I persisted, this time asking, How many times did he get up in the night?

"Three or four," he said.

"Did it hurt?"

"No," he said.

From what he told me, he indicated he had no prostate problem. *Viejos* slept long hours and getting up three or four times in a ten-hour night did not seem too bad to Erazo, although it surely would strike a younger man, with stronger kidneys, to be quite often.

I was not prepared to carry my cursory investigation further, but I did realize that Erazo and other *viejos* ate zinc-rich foods and that zinc is said to be good for the prostate.

Erazo discussed all matters, including his prostate gland and his urinary habits, frankly, easily. His attitude seemed to say, "If you have an interest in my urinary tract, that means you care about me, and that is good. I like that, it pleases me, you make me happy."

Even as open as Erazo had seemed to those friends and loved ones around him, he still had a "past" that haunted him. As we sat along the river bank, he began to uncover a long-buried secret. I felt he was forcing me to practice psychiatry without a license, but I stayed silent, looked off into space, only half listened, interested yet disinterested.

"I have three sons, in Palanda, all of them married, *ya hombres casados . . .*" I was struck not by the meaning of his words, but by his muffled, funereal undertone, like a voice coming from a grave. He was, I knew, coping with a stress in his past and present —by putting that pain on public view. I heard him talking of Huilcopamba, the old original name for the Sacred Valley. He was saying he had another son, and he hated him, hated him enough to kill. Erazo was no longer speaking to me, he was no longer aware that I sat beside him. He was moving his lips, evoking not words so much as suffering and a guilt he had long supported in his heart. I heard him sigh. His voice became lower. He wanted that son to die. I did not interrupt, this moment might be his last opportunity to have said it, once and for all.

The son was born out of wedlock. And he lived across the river. Erazo felt a hatred, an *odio*, for the son and the mother of the son, and worse he felt a self-hatred for the evil he had done them. And now, this incredibly old man in our incredible isolation, was trying somehow to atone for a remembered sin with only a stranger to hear him out.

"I was a brute, *de bruto*," he confessed, his voice an almost inaudible groan.

The evil he had done that mother and his son probably was the greatest stress Erazo had endured, far greater than all of the injustices others had meted out to him. But Erazo was dealing with his stress. He had the gift or talent for forgiveness. Because he could forgive others, he could forgive himself.

Once, Erazo and another *viejo* and I sat drinking coffee and the *viejo*, who claimed he was 105, said that he had led a good life and that when he died he would go to heaven, *el cielo*.

Erazo immediately chimed in, "And I'm going to *el cielo*, too." Then he turned to me, "I asked *Papa Dios* for forgiveness," and he paused, adding rather triumphantly, "And I got it." Erazo saw himself worthy, he found himself "lovable" and saw no reason why *Papa Dios* and the rest of us should not see him that way, also.

One religious injunction has it that we should think on those things that are good, reject those thoughts that are evil. And the *viejos* were artists at finding the good.

Successful aging means accepting the consequences of choices made. The psychologist Erikson speaks of the value of acceptance in the sense that one is able to say, "It was the best life it could have been."

The *viejos* have this kind of acceptance. Given their circumstances, they made the best of life. Mostly, you might have said, it was all in their minds. And saying that, you would have been completely right.

Summation

My approach to the Sacred Valley had elements of fantasy in it. I saw it in my mind's eye where one might live in a pure, guileless, childlike way, free from the primitive emotions of fear and hate, cleansed of environment impurities, close to some heavenly ideal of faith and peace.

But it was an illusion. You and I can never return to that Perfect Place, if indeed it ever existed outside our dreams. We may dream of simplicity, of brotherhood and goodness, of eternal candlelight and togetherness, like Dorothy's Land of Oz. But we cannot return to our origins, as we idealize them. Nor do any of us really desire to "go back"—to live in a mud hut with dirt floors, no running water or inside plumbing.

Still, the *viejos*, living close to nature and still naturally wise and unacquisitive, have much to teach us.

They live certain "truths." The first is the "truth" that health is not a commodity that you can buy at a corner drugstore or get from a high-priced doctor. In our worship of scientific progress, we have come to think that we can turn our bodies over to a doctor, and that he can prescribe some "wonder" drug or perform some "miracle" operation to make us well. We are now learning that doctors—and hospitals—can exacerbate an illness as well as cure it. We are now learning about the dangerous side effects of the drugs many doctors too eagerly prescribe. The *viejos* remind us that health and longevity are basically do-it-yourself propositions.

A second "truth" gleaned from the Sacred Valley: You can live out your life taking care of yourself, dressing yourself, making your own bed, preparing your meals, being self-sufficient. The *viejos* are able to do for themselves as long as they live. You can forget about "retirement" to a rocking chair. If you stop one type of work or activity, you can start anew on other projects, other plans. Take up gardening. Volunteer to help others. Be involved. The *viejos* do not know the meaning of the word "retirement" from activity. He or she has no fear of being warehoused in a nursing home, helpless, degraded, alone and friendless.

A third "truth": You have two "doctors"—your left leg and your right leg. And, while in your lifestyle you won't be climbing el Chaupi with Señor Ramon, you can adopt an exercise program that will keep you younger and greatly prolong your life. As pointed out in chapter 3, your body muscles can easily be rejuvenated with conditioning exercises. And you can have stronger and "younger" muscles at 55 than you had at 15.

Four: You can eat much less beef—and still get all the proteins you need. The *viejos* eat almost *no* beef—they get their proteins from cheese, vegetables, nuts and other sources. They have half the fat content in their blood serum as we Americans. We can do without some of our canned foods with their additives, and eat more "natural," raw foods. Few of us get "a balanced diet"—whatever that is!—and we do need certain supplements, such as vitamin C and vitamin E. It is said that insufficient vitamin C is likely to be the decisive contributing cause when arteries begin to degenerate. A Czech scientist, Dr. Emil Ginter, has found that a daily dose of less than one gram (1,000 mg.) of vitamin C taken over a period of 47 days lowers the blood level of cholesterol by about 10 percent in human beings. Vitamin

E, called the anti-aging pill, helps to protect the body against ozone toxicity and nitrogen dioxide—both ingredients of smog. Since both pesticides and ozone inhibit one enzyme—acetylcholinesterase—vitamin E may protect against the mutual (and perhaps interacting) effect of both toxins.

Also, Dr. Lester Packer of Lawrence Berkeley Laboratory in California has shown that vitamin E retards cell-aging laboratory cell cultures. Normally, human cells divide or redouble about 50 times in laboratory cell cultures. By enriching the fluid in which the cells grow with vitamin E, Dr. Packer has had cells divide more than 200 times, while still retaining the characteristics of young cells.

The *viejos*, eating "pure" fresh foods, with no chemicals, no additives, get their vitamins in natural foods, whereas, we, with our processed foods, need the supplements.

A fifth "truth": You can grow as old as an Erazo but you need not grow senile. The *viejos* met new challenges with each day: to get water up a steep mountain, to grow crops on rocky terrain. You can set your own challenges. Read books and discuss them. Play chess. In his longevity studies at Duke University, Dr. Ewald Busse said that tests show that "those who keep using their brains don't lose their capacity, that a 70 or 80 year old can think as well as anyone, provided he has kept his mind occupied." Here the age-old adage still applies: *use it or lose it*.

In the first seven chapters of this book, I focused on the physical aspects of health and longevity: exercise, environment, diet and habits such as smoking and drinking. Your physical self is your Personality No. 1.

In the final chapters, I focused on the emotional aspects of our lives—the psychological and spiritual forces—or, Personality No. 2.

Many in our pragmatic society have been afraid to deal with Personality No. 2. But it is this side of us that must cope with stress, with the understanding of anger and hate and love, with the enjoyment of our relationships, also with our higher "spiritual" selves.

I found that the *viejos* had reached a remarkable maturation in their development—and integration—of their personalities.

Their psychological and spiritual maturation has aided in their attainment of good health and long life.

Their emotional stability has, I believe, been the most important factor in achieving their longevity.

In our society we have eliminated some of the crudest forms of economic injustice. But we establish many of our priorities and relationships on a basis of aggressive competition and of endless striving for "success." About a million people are hospitalized each year for mental disease and more than ten million are said to be in need of psychiatric treatment. Vascular diseases ruin the heart or brain, and cancers run riot. We have one of the highest rates of any nation for drug addiction and death from violence. And in any one year, it is estimated that more than 17,000 Americans commit suicide.

I did not hear of a single case of a suicide in the Sacred Valley.

The *viejos* could not imagine why those who came to study them put so much emphasis on their years. They had not aspired to old age, nor pursued a regimen to arbitrarily add years to their lives. They were beneficiaries of a mysterious process, and were not concerned about the biology of it. They would look at me disbelievingly when I kept inquiring into possible causes and reasons. I finally realized that they far preferred to talk about the challenge of *today*, rather than the fact that they had defied the actuarial tables.

For the *viejo*, the challenge was dealing with his limitations.

A *viejo*, such as Señor Sanchez, had as much stress as anyone I know, and he met the challenge and dealt with the stress.

"I do the best I can, then I refuse to worry," Señor Sanchez had said.

A *viejo* does not hate, he is not bitter. And by turning off hate, and revenge, he makes himself—or herself—into a figure of broader dimensions, of deeper lovableness, if you will.

These characteristics are important in the light that doctors are now saying that there are psychological characteristics (mistrust of others, bitterness, self-hate, etc.) that *predispose* a person to cancer or bad arteries or to a heart attack. If this is so, it tells us something about our emotional makeup. More than a million people in the United States die of cardiovascular disease, and coronary thrombosis is the leading cause of deaths.

Also it is said that if a man can say he sees a "meaning" in his life he is less likely to get sick than if he feels he is living a lonely, meaningless existence.

Living with "meaning," fulfilling your destiny, does not mean that you must act on a big stage, have a big title or a big salary. That is delusive melodrama. "Meaning" implies purpose of more limited design, living your life, mistakes and all, in the knowledge that it was probably the best that your life, given the circumstances, could have been. This means an acceptance of unfulfillment.

"How had you lived so long?" I asked Carpio.

"Oh," he said, quite simply, "it was my destiny."

He found that simply by living out his destiny he was giving his life a meaning. And believing this, he freed himself of stress, of worries. Many of my sophisticated friends, who seek only material goals, say they feel no sense of "meaning," no sense of fulfillment.

However, millions of Americans now are becoming aware of our need for "quiet" periods, for allowing our lives to be directed by our higher spiritual selves.

As a *viejo* can remind us, we often find "meaning" when we turn inward, to silence.

I once asked Ramon what was the meaning of his

life and he replied quite calmly, "The meaning of life is death." Acceptance of death, for him, meant he could *begin* life anew—each day—free of worry.

I think of him when I see the leaves fall. And I think of him when I see the cherry blossoms along the tidal basin in the nation's capital, proclaiming the "death" of winter, the "birth" of spring. He felt a part of this ongoing cycle of life-in-death, death-in-life. In this sense he is able to eternalize his life, to free himself of worry about his tomorrow, knowing that *Papa Dios* has a plan not only for the trees and the flowers, but for him, as well.

Index

ABOUT THE AUTHOR

GRACE HALSELL was born in west Texas. She has studied at the Sorbonne, has lived and worked in Lima, London, Berlin and Tokyo. Her dispatches for twelve southwestern newspapers, the *New York Herald-Tribune*, and the *New York Post*, have been datelined Russia, Korea and Vietnam. She has lived on a fishing junk in Hong Kong and traveled 2,000 miles down the Amazon by tug. In Washington she was a correspondent covering the Kennedy administration, and was a White House staff writer during the Johnson administration. She is the author of four books for young adults and four adult titles. In 1968 she took a medication to turn her skin black, and lived and worked in Harlem and Mississippi as a black woman. She recorded her experiences in the bestselling *Soul Sister*, published in 1969.

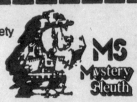

How's Your Health?

Bantam publishes a line of informative books, written by top experts to help you toward a healthier and happier life.

☐	10350	**DR. ATKINS' SUPERENERGY DIET,** Robert Atkins, M.D.	$2.25
☐	2111	**FASTING: The Ultimate Diet,** Allan Cott, M.D.	$1.75
☐	11287	**WEIGHT CONTROL THROUGH YOGA,** Richard Hittleman	$1.75
☐	11872	**A DICTIONARY OF SYMPTOMS,** Gomez	$2.25
☐	6417	**THE BRAND NAME NUTRITION COUNTER,** Carper	$1.95
☐	7602	**SWEET AND DANGEROUS,** John Yudkin, M.D.	$1.95
☐	7709	**NUTRITION AGAINST DISEASE,** Roger J. Williams	$1.95
☐	7793	**NUTRITION AND YOUR MIND,** George Watson	$1.95
☐	11589	**THE NEW AEROBICS,** Kenneth Cooper, M.D.	$1.95
☐	11628	**AEROBICS FOR WOMEN,** Kenneth Cooper, M.D.	$1.95
☐	11412	**THE ALL-IN-ONE CARBOHYDRATE GRAM COUNTER,** Jean Carper	$1.75
☐	10175	**WHICH VITAMINS DO YOU NEED?** Martin Ebon	$1.95
☐	12107	**WHOLE EARTH COOKBOOK,** Cadwallader and Ohr	$1.95
☐	10865	**FASTING AS A WAY OF LIFE,** Allan Cott, M.D.	$1.75
☐	11292	**THE ALL-IN-ONE CALORIE COUNTER,** Jean Carper	$1.75
☐	11402	**THE FAMILY GUIDE TO BETTER FOOD AND BETTER HEALTH,** Ron Deutsch	$2.25

Buy them at your local bookstore or use this handy coupon for ordering:

Bantam Books, Inc., Dept. HN, 414 East Golf Road, Des Plaines, Ill. 60016

Please send me the books I have checked above. I am enclosing $_____ (please add 50¢ to cover postage and handling). Send check or money order —no cash or C.O.D.'s please.

Mr/Mrs/Miss_____

Address_____

City_____State/Zip_____

HN—7/78

Please allow four weeks for delivery. This offer expires 1/79.

Bantam Book Catalog

Here's your up-to-the-minute listing of every book currently available from Bantam.

This easy-to-use catalog is divided into categories and contains over 1400 titles by your favorite authors.

So don't delay—take advantage of this special opportunity to increase your reading pleasure.

Just send us your name and address and 25¢ (to help defray postage and handling costs).